3205

BOOK No. 38392
UNIVERSITY OF BIRMINGHAM EXTRAMURAL LIBRARY

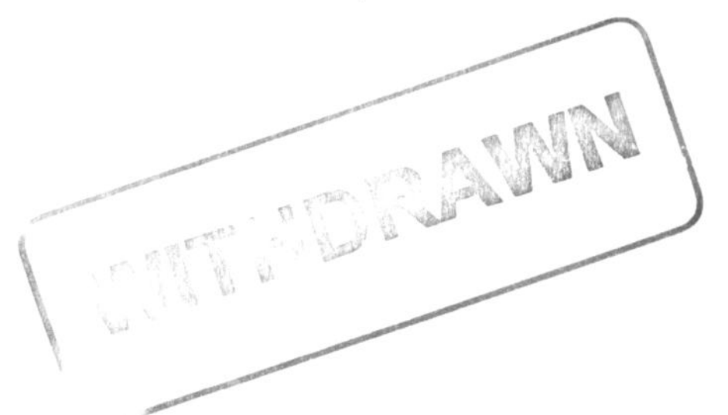

My Brother's Keeper?

Second Edition

Monnica C. Stewart
MB, BS, D (Obst) RCOG

*Assistant Physician, Geriatric Department,
Edgware General Hospital, Middlesex*

FOREWORD
by
William Evans
MD, DSc, FRCP

HEALTH HORIZON LIMITED
Publishers for
THE CHEST AND HEART ASSOCIATION
Tavistock House North, London, WC1H 9JE

First edition published July 1968
Second edition published January 1971

TO DOUGLAS AND EV RITCHIE

The perfect team, not only of husband and wife, but also of 'stroke' patient and supporting relative. The generosity with which they have shared their experiences and achievements has helped countless disabled people throughout the world to lead fuller and richer lives.

This book is published by
Health Horizon Limited
for
The Chest and Heart Association
Tavistock House North, Tavistock Square, London, WC1H 9JE
and printed by Waterlow and Sons Ltd., London and Dunstable

© Monnica C. Stewart, MB, BS, D(Obst) RCOG 1970

SBN 901548 18 9

CONTENTS

ACKNOWLEDGEMENTS

The writer of a first book requires much support and encouragement. I have received more than my just meed, both professionally and domestically. So much so that it seems invidious to single out names.

Any failure to 'communicate' remains my sole responsibility. If I succeed, my debt to my team of helpers is redoubled. Particularly so to Mrs. Margaret B. Hawker, who toiled long hours over the editing with me and who produced the diagrams, together with Mrs. Gillian Gadsden. To Mrs. Florence Vincent and Miss Marilyn Wilmshurst, who laboured so thoughtfully over their typewriters. Dr. Madeleine Eggleston, Mrs. Lynette Farmer, Mrs. Janet Rabson, and Miss Dorothy Thomas, gave much constructive advice. And not least, to my publishers, *Health Horizon Limited*—and Dr. Harley Williams, from whom came the original idea. Also Miss Hilda Walsh and her colleagues who have steered me through the intricacies of publication.

Finally, I acknowledge my abiding gratitude to my patients, their relatives and friends. Without their tolerant training and the distilled wisdom of Dr. F. Allen Binks—this book would never have come to life.

FOREWORD

This is not just another book, not one written primarily for the enjoyment of the reader, nor the aggrandisement of the author, but one intended to give pain, inviting sympathy, to those who will acquaint themselves of the pathos which the author meets unendingly in her daily work as she struggles to patch the broken lives of her patients. Her heart is in this work, and her words come from the heart; they form a prayer that those both within and outside her profession should come urgently to her aid. She speaks from the premise that it is not so much the disease process that proves a hindrance to a healthy equilibrium, but the adverse situations in which patients find themselves.

Medicine has two primary avowed objects, to discover the nature of a patient's illness, and to heal him. The doctor reaches the first objective through his clinical sense, sometimes helped by laboratory tests. The second he achieves through prescribing one or more of only a dozen medicaments of proven worth; occasionally he summons surgery to his aid. His work, however, is incomplete and effete if he has left unrepaired any injury which prohibits his patient from leading an independent existence, and if he fails to uplift a faltered spirit or allay a disturbed mind. To enable a patient to meet the handicap of a residual physical disability, resuscitate his lost self-reliance, and maintain an equable mental stability in the face of diverse frustrations is a goal to achieve before a doctor lays claim to the accolade of therapeutic success.

The convalescing period following an illness is illness no less. Indeed, this final phase of the illness often requires greater thought and attention from the attending physician than that demanded when symptoms are most prominent, for although the period of medicinal therapy may have been concluded, restitution to normal health is so often delayed for a variable time.

In the case of elderly people the majority die at home and a high proportion of these have suffered from prolonged indisposition before their demise. Whatever the nature of their illness, they bear it with commendable patience, and often with shining courage, so that the outside world and even their friends and near relatives are not made aware of their suffering. Old age by itself is sickness enough, but when organic disease is added, to live an independent existence may be no longer possible, when help from outside is solicited. It is then that the family physician finds that he has inadequate time to devote to such a house-bound or bed-bound patient, and seeks help elsewhere, usually admitting her or him to hospital where a stay can only be for a short time. Too many frail and elderly people are herded into Old People's Homes. It should be for the Welfare State and Society to help these worthy folk to live on in their own homes. Such preferential treatment is owing to them because on their shoulders the present generation was raised. The National Health Service should turn urgently to succour this class of needy elderly who are suffering in our midst.

WILLIAM EVANS,
MD, DSc, FRCP

Consulting Physician, Cardiac Department,
The London Hospital, National Heart Hospital
and Institute of Cardiology, London

June 1968

PREFACE TO SECOND EDITION

When the stock of the first edition was running low, my publishers asked me to consider the form of Mark II. I set about the task gladly and I expected there would be much to alter.

It was sobering to discover that so little of a tangible nature had happened to the Geriatric Department between December 1967 and August 1970. And so the book stands as it did, except that two more chapters have been added.

This has been a period of intense but intangible activity for us. We have been participants in many discussions and meetings both locally and farther afield. We have taken part in training programmes of all kinds. We have written many words in many publications. We have battled ceaselessly to try and stem the swamping tide and turn it into more productive channels.

In these endeavours we have been fortunate to be supported by a keen and slightly augmented paramedical staff and by a magnificent corps of reablists. This is the most heartening feature of "the years between". The reablists are being recognised in their own right as the people on whom the patients and the professionals depend to produce for the patients a quality of support so sadly lacking in institutional living.

The reablists are indeed the community coming in, the commonsense housewife and mother (or father!) providing the personal touch of continuity, warmth and the contact point that the professionals now have too little time to supply.

The description of a reablist's work would require a book in itself. Meanwhile I salute our reablists and offer to our vital "continuity" women and men, past and present, the dedication of the extra part of Mark II.

London, August 1970.

ACKNOWLEDGEMENTS FOR SECOND EDITION

As the second edition goes to print it becomes even more obvious how vital team work is in all aspects of life. I may be the person who actually dips the pen in the ink, but the thoughts expressed have been hammered largely on the anvil of discussion with my colleagues and friends. To them I am indebted.

Once more I would like to record my gratitude to Mrs. Florence Vincent for her cheerful help with the typing. To Mrs. Margaret Hawker for her ungrudging help with editing and also to Mr. John Tripp for his constructive criticism and practical semantic help.

To my friends and colleagues at home and at work I have even greater cause to offer thanks for support, for between editions I have experienced personally some of the dilemmas of the working daughter.

As always the final word of thanks must go to the publishers and printers, without whose guidance and patience no author can be more than sounding brass or tinkling symbol.

INTRODUCTION

This book is a *cri du coeur* from a hard-pressed Geriatric Department that has been squeezed to its limits and now the veritable pips are beginning to squeak.

"The buck stops here " said Harry S. Truman, and those with whom it stops, such as our particular Geriatric Unit at Edgware General Hospital, recognise that inevitably and inexorably we will be driven into a corner.

The day never dawns without there coming one more request for help with '*the disposal*' of yet another elderly occupant of a bed, residing either *at* home or in a *Home*, or in a hospital. Yearly, the explosion of the pensionable population becomes more shattering. Like the atom bomb, this is a previously unexperienced phenomenon. (*Figures* 1*a*, 1*b and* 1*c—see page* 8). The consequence of the passing of the National Health Service Act of 1948 ensured the abolition of the penal relegation aspects of the Poor Law, but twenty years on, the effects of the Poor Law's authoritarian and imperative approach still linger, and underlie much of the thought or action connected with the terms 'Chronic Sick', 'Incurable', 'Geriatric' or 'Long Stay'.

In the 1900s, when the proportion of pensionable population was 1 : 21, the problem of disposal of the frail, infirm aged was simple; it was only deemed necessary to provide a stark building, put in iron bedsteads and small wooden lockers* and fill to capacity and over. None could be rejected and none needed to be. All that was required was provision of shelter from the cruder elements, clothing and food and custodians to cope with bed care. Standards were abysmal outside. The workhouse could have seemed palatial to many and there were always workers available to provide the custodianship. The idea seemed to be, put simply, that for those for whom there was nothing to do, nothing was needed to do it with.

*Norton, Doreen. "*Hospitals of the Long-Stay Patient*" (1967). *Chapter VII*, 3.11. "Rather surprisingly, not all hospitals appeared to have a bedside locker for every patient. Eight either declined to answer or their reply was not specific but five indicated that they did not have enough, one of these specifying the reason as being 'due to lack of space between beds'."

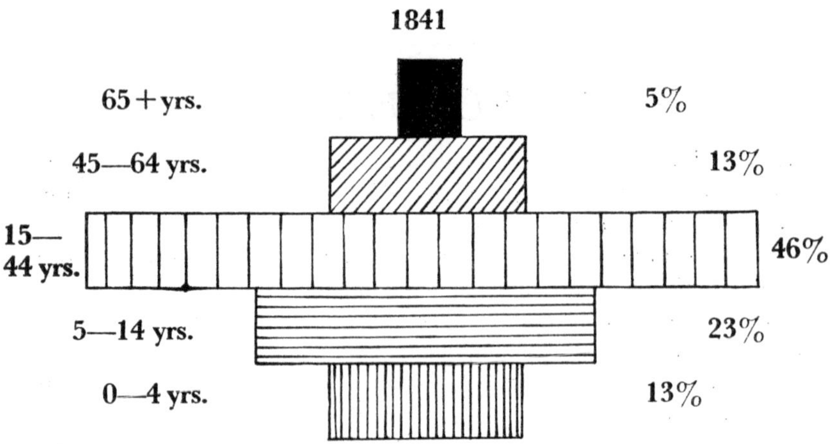

1841
65 + yrs.
5%
45—64 yrs.
13%
15—44 yrs.
46%
5—14 yrs.
23%
0—4 yrs.
13%

Figure 1a

1901
65 + yrs.
8%
45—64 yrs.
15%
15—44 yrs.
45%
5—14 yrs.
21%
0—4 yrs.
11%

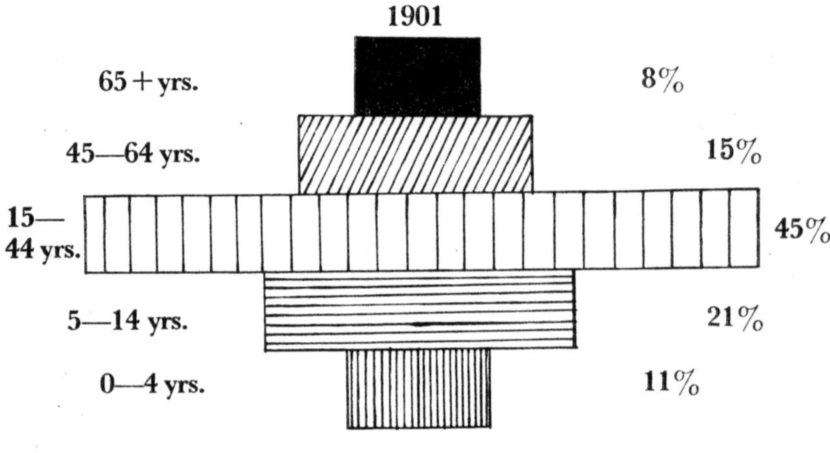

Figure 1b

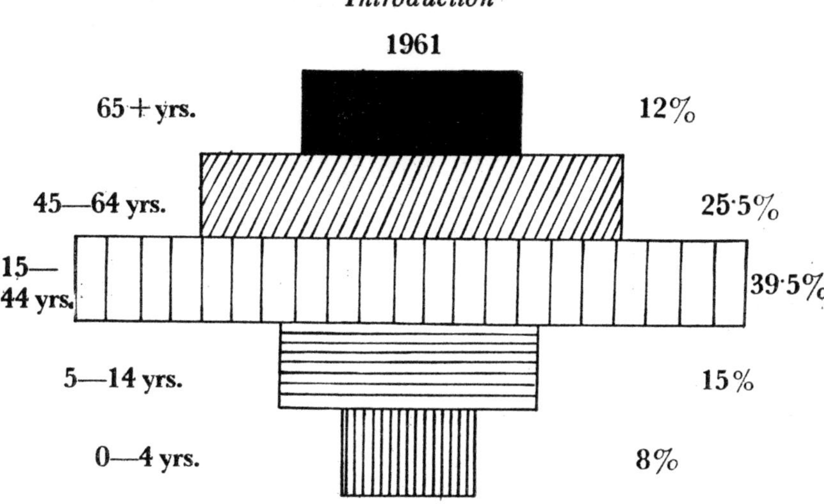

Figure 1c

Have things altered? In the 1970s, with the proportion of those over 65 up to 1 : 5 (*Figure* 2—*see page* 10) and the standard of living incomparably higher for the general population, the statutory accommodation for the elderly is fast becoming intolerable. There is no specific apparatus or technique for 'disposing' of people. There are no longer any 'human warehouses' with elastic walls where people can be stored until death takes them. What is needed—which, for some obscure reason seems to be a scarce commodity, is a genuine desire to support people in difficulty, with all the knowledge, individual skills and facilities available, until such time as they can regain as much independence as possible for personal living and once more have dignity as "sophisticated adults".[1]

To do this requires not so much technical skill and professional expertise as an adequate clinical philosophy, human understanding, basic common sense and a willingness to become involved and accept responsibility.

Every moment brings us nearer to crisis point, and "*Sans Everything*"[2] will only be a precursor of the explosions and implosions that will rock the conscience of the community, unless the community becomes alive to the danger and takes crash action to re-think and plan ahead.

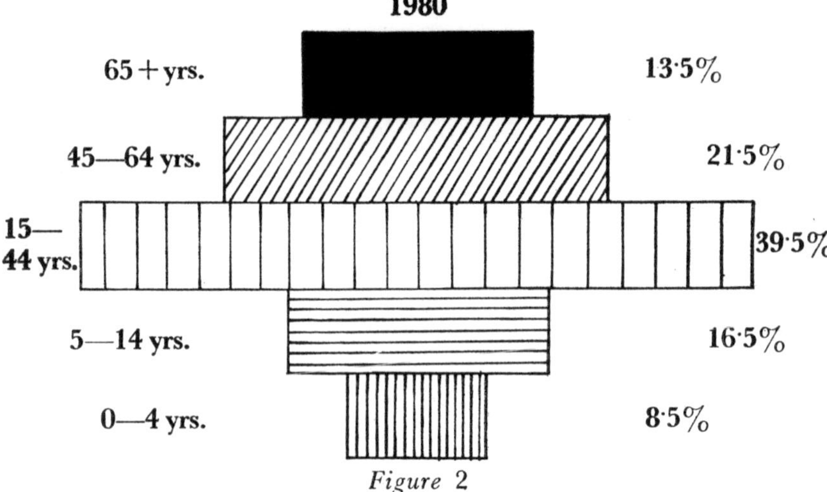

Figure 2

We with whom the 'buck stops' are finding ourselves with less and less room to manoeuvre. We are being driven into a corner but we feel strongly that it is best to be driven into the neatest corner possible; we therefore try and look ahead and around and out—as far and as wide as the human eye can see and the imagination stretch. Anything goes; parataxis is rampant. There is no order, no pattern, few precedents and no blueprints for us to follow. It is a groping forward across unknown country, uncharted territory. This has never happened before in recorded history. No civilisation has known an explosion of population in the over sixties range previously.

This must be understood.
This must be accepted.

The old shibboleths are as meaningful as the mutterings of incantations to the moon.

Firstly, I will outline some of our problems, and then I will try and trace how our lines of thought and action have developed in an endeavour to cope with these problems. Basically, we undertake a dual function—palliation and, if possible, dynamic solution of the problems in the here and now—and at the same time making a furious prophylactic effort to prevent such problems occurring and recurring in the future.

Once one moves into the paths of prevention, one leaves safe charted routes, hallowed by time and convention, and one encounters Stygian labyrinths and embarks on troubled seas.

Given a staunch captain and a good crew, this voyage can be a challenge of infinite excitement and discovery. There can be immense satisfaction in seeing just one person arising from a bedfast hulk of rejected misery into a state of social competence once more.

Chance and random development—the haphazardness of the typical British no-planning—have gone into making the physical properties of our Unit what they are today. We are the heirs of the Poor Law boundaries of 1895. We are, in a sense, more fortunate than many of our colleagues up and down the country, for *we* have not inherited the old workhouse infirmary. That honour falls to the Welfare Department of one of the three Greater London Boroughs that bound us. The old workhouse is now a 'Home' (*sic*) for 245.

Instead, we have a motley collection of ex-isolation hospitals, old isolated country houses and 'temporary' structures from the 1914-18 War—these in nine different places in a 45-square mile area. (*Figure* 3 *see page* 12).

Figure 4 (*see page* 13) relates the population at risk—the national estimated hospital bed requirement—compared with the actual numbers allocated.

It becomes clear immediately that quantitatively, the needs are being met only half way. When one proceeds to qualitative comparisons, then the imagination boggles. One can only wonder anew at the devotion of the staff involved in the running of these annexes which have such limited provision for civilised living. One marvels at the *esprit de corps* and cheerful resourcefulness in overcoming, or ignoring, so many hindrances and drawbacks.*

*Norton, Doreen. "*Hospitals of the Long-Stay Patient*" (1967). *Chapter XII,* 4.50. "Service before self is paramount—this being exemplified in the Matron. Indeed, it seems that those who, unconditionally, choose to work in long stay hospitals can only be one of two things—saints or fools—for none but a saint or a fool would elect to spend a working life in this environment. All the more reason, then, that the service they give to a large section of the chronically ill and aged community be matched by an equally high standard in working conditions and in tools for the task."

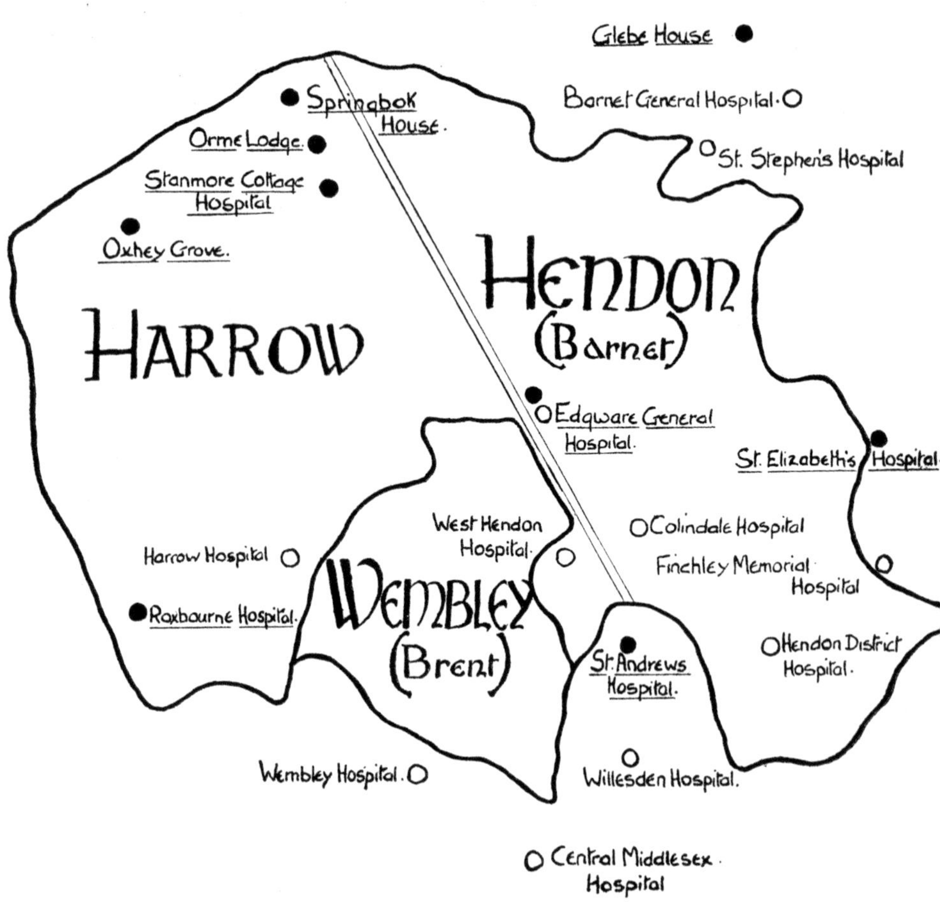

● Geriatric Hospitals

○ Other Hospitals

Figure 3

Overall Population of area—*see map page* 12	...	**455,000**
Over 65 years	...	**52,000**
Recommended No. Hospital Beds— (1 bed per 100 over 65 years)	...	**520**

Actual Beds—

	Male	*Female*
Edgware General Hospital ...	20	18
Roxbourne Hospital	14	38
Oxhey Grove		30
Orme Lodge		22
Stanmore Cottage Hospital ...		14
St. Elizabeth's Hospital		23
Glebe House		24
Springbok House	← 15 →	
St. Andrew's Hospital	15	12
	TOTAL	245

Figure 4

A dominant factor is that only 38 of the 245 beds available are in a purpose built hospital and these are the only beds with the expected facilities of a general district hospital. But as each annexe has developed its own special atmosphere, one of the cardinal human needs *can* be met—there is variability of choice in both the location and the particular character of each place, and it is rare to the point of exception to be unable to find an accepting niche for even the most difficult personality.

One is reminded of a passage, reported from a speech made by Sir George Godber (Chief Medical Officer of the Ministry of Health) at an Annual Conference of the *National Association of Mental Health* in 1966 :

"The hospital service took over some 3,000 separate hospital units. Most of them were small; many of them were ancient; it is fair to say that none of them had the structure, equipment or function of the hospital of the future. One tenth of that number of well-planned, properly located district hospitals would provide almost all the hospital and specialist care for the future."

And there is the rub. Ten-year hospital plans seem to have been on the table for many years. Always we seem to be marking time, awaiting the millennium. Radical changes and alterations are shelved as uneconomical, when all is to be so different in the Brave New World visualised in the ten-year plan. One could paraphrase Stephen Leacock's explanation of electricity:

"Plans are two kinds—positive and negative. The difference is, I presume, that one comes a little more expensive but is more durable; the other is a cheaper thing but the moths get into it."[3]

And this is why there is little point in kicking against the pricks. One must accept what cannot be changed but always retain enough strength to improve, whenever and whatever possible. Even if actual buildings cannot be altered, at least the environment within these structures can be made more civilised for all the people living and working within them. The word strength is used advisedly, as it requires constant vigilance to prevent the drug of apathy dulling awareness of purpose. There has to be not only a profound clinical and social philosophy; it is essential to have colleagues of like mind, always questioning, so that if one should falter despondently, others can maintain the corporate morale.

At Edgware General Hospital, in the Geriatric Department, our particular clinical and social philosophy has become more a way of life, and it has evolved slowly over the years. It is never easy to categorise how things come about, but if one reads three articles: "The Functions of a Hospital",[4] "Background to Disability",[5] "The Approach to Disability and Breakdown"[6] together with the Report of the Standing Conference for Old People's Welfare (Greater London) on the Care of Infirm Old People,[7] one can sense the personality and thought progressions of our Medical Director, Dr. F. Allen Binks; from him stems the general attitude in the department as a whole. Dr. Binks has an unerring instinct, as Churchill was once described[8] as having, for getting to the heart of the matter—an essential ability in his thinking which cuts through all the dead wood of accepted practice which inhibits any kind of progress. He can peel away the layers of habitual thought like a chef peeling an onion. This is real discrimination, which is so much more valuable than the automatic acceptance of anything new and the facile rejection of anything old.

The credo of the department has been summarised succinctly in "The Approach to Disability and Breakdown".

> **"It is a matter of trying to enable many people, some not very well equipped, to live effective and fulfilling lives as independently as possible for a normal life span of some 70 to 80 years or more, with all the difficulties this involves.**
>
> **This has never had to be done before to the extent now demanded of us . . .**
>
> **The technical treatment of disease processes alone is quite inadequate. . . .**
>
> **It is not the offence of destitution which must concern us . . . but the breakdown in effective and independent living and the place the hospital has in trying to rectify this, bearing in mind the fact that the greatest difficulties centre around those who, for one reason or another, lack the reserves or the response to regain personal independence."[9]**

Another way of saying this is to point out that the traditional method of applying the battery of all known mechanico-clinical techniques and investigations to people and then discharging them from hospital when these are complete, is not working any more. This approach will not of itself restore people to health and independence. Doing this *to*, rather than *with* people, will seldom achieve the desired results. Society is no longer able to contain the failures and rejects produced by this system. The family and the chronic sick hospital—the long accepted containing repository for custodial care—are disappearing fast, and we are being left with the swamp of older people, handicapped and not able to maintain independence independently.

Re-mobilisation—re-activation for its own sake—is not enough. It is only a short-term policy. Problems of retirement, social isolation, boredom, rejection or even over-solicitude, produce a slow draining of morale unless fulfilment can be found within the person's own creative effort, his own company or his own home. Housing, welfare and community services are not yet adequately or foresightedly geared. History has never had an equivalent situation; no civilisation has ever had an elderly population of such magnitude, and these older people have to be able to find reasons for living.

> "Tho' much is taken, much abides; and tho'
> we are not now that strength which in old days
> moved earth and Heaven; that which we are, we are."
>
> *Tennyson*

References

1. Ritchie, Douglas. (1961). *Proceedings of The Chest and Heart Association Symposium on 'Stroke' Rehabilitation*. Guildhall, London.
2. Robb, Barbara. (1967). "*Sans Everything—A Case to Answer.*" London. *Nelson. Price* 18*s*. 0*d*.
3. Leacock, Stephen. (1910). "*Literary Lapses—A Manual of Education.*"
4 Binks, F. Allen. (1962). *Lancet,* **i,** 1083-86.
5. *Ibidem.* (1964), **ii,** 1233-36.
6. Binks, F. Allen. (1968). *Brit. Med. J.*, **i,** 269-74.
7. *The Care of Infirm Old People*. Report of a Study Group of the Standing Conference for Old People's Welfare (Gt. London), 1966.
8. H.R.H. Duke of Edinburgh. (1964). *Address at opening of Churchill College, Cambridge.*
9. Binks, F. Allen. (1968). *Brit. Med. J.*, **i,** 269-74.

Chapter One

STROKE

"Bearing in mind the fact that the greatest difficulties centre around those who for one reason or another lack the reserves or the response to reach personal independence . . ." [1]

What is basic personal independence?

We postulate this to be: (*Figure* 5—*see* ***page*** 18).

The ability:

1) To get in and out of a bed or chair.
2) To move to or from lavatory or commode and manage there.
3) To wash.
4) To dress.
5) To eat.

} UNAIDED

This is basic personal independence, and with time and effort, coupled with professional know-how and adequate incentive (meaning personal desire to regain independence), there should be few who are not able to achieve such a goal. If to this can be added the ability to climb stairs, get in and out of a car and do some domestic chores, then life has added savour.

It is strange how little is taught to doctors and the paramedical staff in their training about the need for incentive. Text books abound in description of how miracles may be wrought—by application of surgical techniques, use of complex apparatus or exhibition of potent drugs, but never is mention made of a need to find a motivating response within the patient. Acquiescence appears to be all that is expected of him, and compliance. If, despite all, he stubbornly refuses either to get better or to die but instead continues to occupy a hospital bed, then a breakdown of relationships between the patient and the hospital staff may easily ensue and he becomes a '*case for disposal*'.

BASIC PERSONAL INDEPENDENCE

= The ability to :—

1) Get in and out of bed or chair

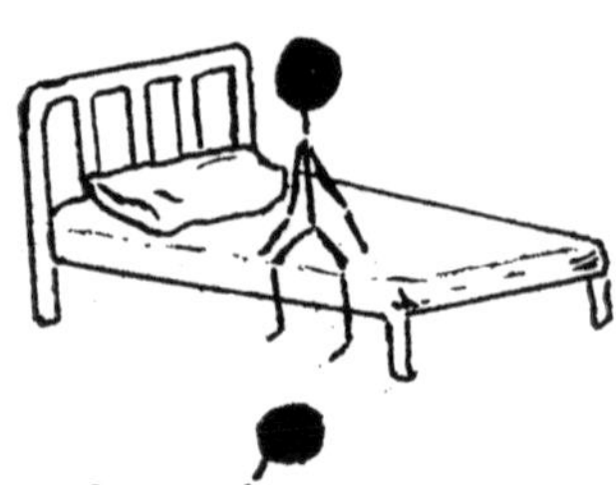

2) Walk to and from the lavatory
(and manage there)

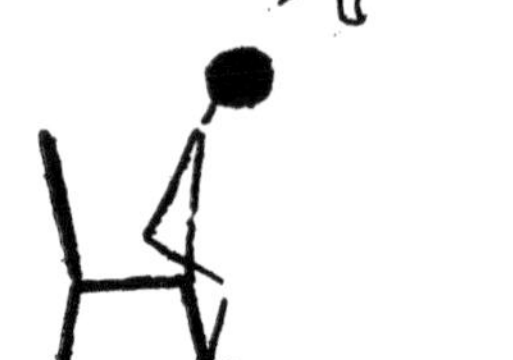

3) Wash

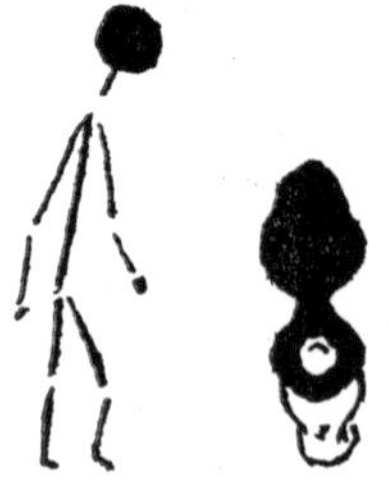

4) Dress

5) Eat

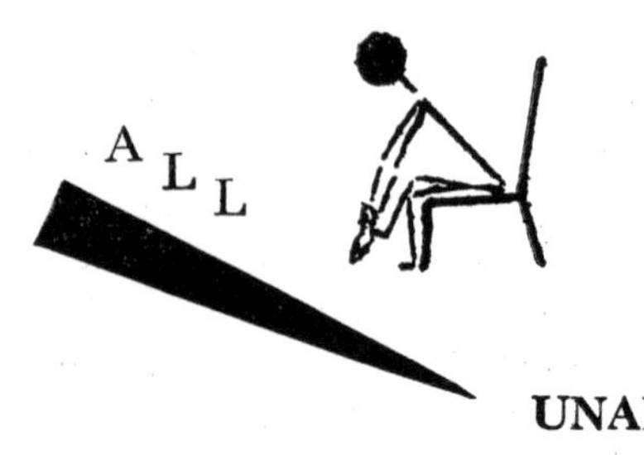

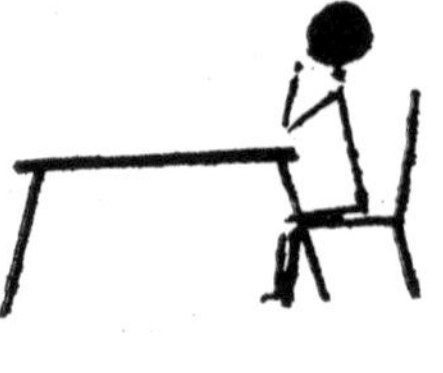

UNAIDED

Figure 5

One of the clearest stories of the battle to return to personal independence is chronicled in Douglas Ritchie's book "*Stroke. A Diary of Recovery*",[2] first published in 1960 but brought up to date by the author in 1965, ten years after his paralysing stroke which also rendered him speechless—a devastating blow to a man whose professional business was words and communication. He was only 50 at the time of his stroke and he was head of BBC publicity. During the war he had been famous and his voice a great solace to friends in occupied Europe, with his 'Colonel Britton' broadcasts.

Douglas Ritchie's story makes horrifying reading nowadays. A position of some social significance, reasonable economic conditions and influential medical acquaintances were apparently of little benefit to him or his wife. The road they had to travel was obscure, rough and ill signposted—seemingly. They had to work out their own route and even make their own maps, very little information being available or being made known to them.

Douglas Ritchie's subsequent writings and speeches have changed things a great deal. He relied on American books and leaflets but following his stirring plea for information for the British patient and relative at *The Chest and Heart Association* Symposium on "Stroke Rehabilitation" held in the Guildhall, London, in June, 1961, there has been a torrent of literature produced in this country which must be helping a considerable number of people.

Douglas Ritchie had two incalculable assets—one, his own dogged courage and determination to return to personal independence and full living, and the other, his wife, who was insistent that "he should not be left to die or live like a vegetable". Without her untiring support and unflagging persistence in finding professional help, it would have taken even someone of Douglas Ritchie's fantastic calibre longer than four years to regain independent living after such a devastating cerebral catastrophe.

The sudden death of Douglas Ritchie in December, 1967, has left the world an emptier but richer place. The obituaries all laid stress on his contribution to the war effort in 1939-45; his stroke and recovery were only mentioned briefly. As Mrs. Ritchie has commented, the work he did after his stroke "was the really hard big thing in his life—the papers dwelled so much on the war-time part—when it was easy to act big—his triumph, his immortal triumph, was to cope with all the littlenesses of recovery and then be so unselfishly constructive and helpful to other 'strokes' ".[3]

Many people of many countries owe a great debt to this man who, in Sir Francis Williams' valedictory words, was so much "a man for all seasons". For us it was a great privilege to have known him and to have had his inspiration and help in our work.

Other cases within one's own clinical purlieu come to mind. *MR. DRIVER,* striken whilst at work in a remote country area and consigned to a chronic sick ward bed for two years, from which he was never moved. Brought from there, by an act of faith on the part of his recently married second wife and stepson, to a new house in an urban area, he was remobilised by his family's efforts and with the guidance of a nearby Physiotherapy Clinic which he attended as an out-patient.

His drive to recovery was such that even two years' immobility could not quench it, but the story has not the triumphant ending of Douglas Ritchie's, for much more is needed than physical remobilisation. This man was also incontinent of urine and faeces. The first was dealt with by the provision of a rubber urinal but the second caused a breakdown in personal relationship with his stepson in whose house they lived, and it was at this stage that we became involved.

And here we must digress a little to explain the procedure. As in many other Geriatric Departments up and down the country (there are 156 at present), it is our policy to try and see every patient before admitting him to one of our hospital beds. This can be done best by one of the team of doctors paying a visit to the patient, be he at home, in an institution or even in another hospital ward. The reasons for this are many; but briefly, in the process of making as full a clinical and social assessment as possible, one establishes contact with the patient as a person; a very salient point when so many elderly people are filled with natural dread and foreboding of hospital admission. Many view it as a process of 'being put away' and fear that once in hospital, there they will remain until death do them part. Some of this apprehension can be ameliorated by the visiting physician's obvious concern for the patient as a person with individual needs. In addition, it is also possible to make a fairly clear estimation of any type of domestic tension; particularly noting interpersonal relationships and whether goodwill remains or whether it has run out permanently.

If goodwill remains, then assessment of environment, such as steps and stairs, position of w.c., running water and general hazards can be made to assist in planning the extent of the re-ablement programme. No person is admitted to one of our beds (except in dire emergency) without there first being formulated a programme of action which will be made known to all who will be concerned with his future welfare. Usually these plans are also made known to the patient and his relatives and discussed with them at the time of the visit, thus helping to prevent any suggestion of conspiracy.

These are vital elements as the physical constraints of the Unit determine that there are three admitting bases, all with differing facilities, and an ongoing plan is essential although, of course, it may require modification according to the person's need after admission.

Lastly, a domiciliary visit is vital to establish priority of admission. The policy of first request, first admission, would be valueless in view of the limited number of beds available and the diversity of facility of the admitting hospitals. It is interesting to note that of every five people seen at home, on an average, only two require admission.

With this explanation of some of the reasons for carrying out domiciliary visiting, let us return to the story of Mr. Driver, who was visited at home at the request of his family doctor. He was found in immaculate surroundings, miserably smoking and fully dressed, but only too well aware that he was a nuisance and very anxious to be admitted to hospital once more, in an endeavour to deal with his incontinence.

Suffice it to say treatment was found to be possible, firstly by dealing surgically with a prostatic enlargement and removing some stones from his bladder. Secondly, by ensuring that his bowels worked regularly and fully, so that his bowel incontinence could be controlled. By adaptation of his clothing and a change of sartorial habit (e.g. wearing a woollen cardigan instead of a suit jacket and elasticising his trouser waist band), he was enabled to be independent for his own dressing needs. The putting on of his caliper shoe remained the only manoeuvre for which help was sometimes required. This was not enough, however, for here was a man who had always worked hard, wagon, tractor or lorry driving. He had little or no intellectual resource and no inclination towards learning any one-handed occupation or skill. He wanted to be at home with his wife but she had to be the breadwinner and he had therefore been left alone and idle for long hours at a stretch. Apart from this, the owner of the house, his stepson, no longer wished to receive him, the initial goodwill having given out long since under the stress of the incontinence and the strain and resentment of seeing his mother chained to this situation.

Here one can visualise the cry going up—that relatives do not honour their obligations and that this is a typical example of an irresponsible family. But is it? When one analyses what has gone into the making of this situation; how little support this family had in the crucial early years after the stroke and how an almost intolerable situation had been supported for so long without complaint, one marvels instead at human endurance.

Now one meets the hard cold facts of divided loyalties and economic provisions head-on. The wife is willing and anxious to have her husband at home with her but she knows she can no longer impose this strain on her son. Economically, whatever small savings she had are gone into the house and she therefore cannot obtain alternative private accommodation, nor does she merit many 'points' in order to receive any priority for council housing. Therefore, the man himself has little option but to acquiesce in accepting the only alternative to continued hospital support—namely, admission to one of the local Welfare Old People's Homes. A devastating decision for all concerned.

At one time we had hoped that, by arranging regular visits home for the day and perhaps in time, for the night and then one or two days, re-acceptance might have occurred; but it has become clear that this will never be so. The only hope will be for the wife to move out of the area to a new satellite town where she may be able to obtain accommodation more rapidly; where, too, lives one of this man's own children who would be able to give more support, though not accommodation. This means, however, that instead of being able to visit frequently, as she is now doing, during the week, with the man returning home for a day during the week-end, there will be lengthy periods of separation. What a trap to be caught in.

Yet, although much of the difficulty has been produced by lack of supporting facilities in the communities in which they have lived to date, some of it is brought about by the particular personality of the man himself; his unwillingness to accept one-handed work, however trivial, in order to find some purpose again in living, is a very potent element in negativism.

What a contrast to the ex-soldier, *MR. ATKINS,* with a left mid-upper arm amputation during the war, who suffered a severe cerebro-vascular accident years after which deprived him of the use of his speech and his right arm and leg. An indomitable optimist, he set about making himself as independent as he possibly could. Whereas before he had spurned a 'hook', he got fitted up with a prosthesis on the left arm as soon as he could and shortly after was learning to write left-handed, performing incredible feats with his hook. When he regained walking power with the aid of a below-knee iron, and whilst his wife was at work, he stumped up to the Occupational Therapy Department on foot. There, his very presence was a vast source of encouragement to older and often less handicapped men. With the aid of all sorts of gadgetry, he obtained a remarkable degree of personal independence. Over the years he has regained a good range of speech and always he has shown unflinching courage and cheerfulness, so that the professionals willingly spend hours planning sources of help for him, without any feeling of exasperation or resentment.

Comparisons may be odious but they are certainly interesting; the more one compares and experiences, the more one comes to realise that sheer technical expertise is of no value unless it is matched by adequate incentive and willingness on the part of the recipient.

To illustrate this even more cogently, there is the incredible *MRS. CRIER* who, one feels, is going to require the indefinite hospitality of hospital support. Mrs. Crier has a simple but common story. One day she and her husband woke up in the bed-sitting room they had, upstairs, at the back of their daughter's house, to find that she had a complete left hemiplegia. She was admitted that day as an emergency to an 'acute' hospital bed. She remained there for nine months, and some of the comments on the notes about her at that time make interesting reading. Because she failed to rehabilitate in a manner consistent with her return of physical capability, the opinion of a psychiatrist was sought. He commented that she appeared to be depressed by her surroundings! As she expressed paranoid ideas against the nurses, it was thought that there was a psychotic element in her depression. Tranquillisers were prescribed but six months later it was noted that she was as noisy and difficult as ever and that her progress on the physical side had been very slow. A firm prescription was made that she must be "forced to walk as she had adequate power". Ultimately the caliper that had been prescribed for her was delivered and she was discharged home to her family the same day.

Fifteen days later a request was made to the Geriatric Department for admission as the patient was incontinent and the family were unable to manage, and the ward from which she had been discharged had refused to have her back again. Her picture was rather confused by the fact that she was still attending, as an out-patient, three times a week for physiotherapy. However, it was at once obvious from the home visit that the family were completely unable to cope with this situation and she was admitted to one of our beds—a miserable failure and totally rejected on all sides. It was realised that she had been rejected from the other ward because she was a failure "for whom no more could be done". We hoped that with acceptance of her as she was, as a person, and with the gradual infiltration of a sense of security, response would emerge and constructive work could begin. Even if she could no longer walk, at least she could achieve some independence and mobility from a wheel-chair. At no time has this been so. All the time there has been demand for treatment to 'cure' her, by either medicine or physiotherapy exercises. The patient and her family have been unceasing and unswerving in their demands for prolonged exercise treatment such as "she had been having in the other ward". Here is an excellent example of the results of relegation to a ward with fewer staff and fewer facilities. The increased demands by the rejected, to compensate for the unfairness of the relegation, add intolerable burdens to the limited staff who are already dealing with multiple problems of a similar nature.

If pondering on what had gone into the making of this particular problem makes it understandable now, one wonders if the facts would have been recognised had similar pains been taken at an earlier stage. There was a practically insoluble domestic situation at home (a breakdown in marital relations, with strong incentive against making *any* recovery to personal independence) and attempts to force recovery by applying techniques to the patient would not have been made. Mrs. Crier's social situation is such that her only release is in either death or indefinite occupation of a hospital bed. If the latter could have been offered to her at a much earlier stage, one suspects that a great deal of the abrasiveness of her personal relationships and those of her family with members of the staff would have been smoothed.

We shall meet other illustrations of 'stroke' patients as we go on, and one imagines that ultimately writer and reader will agree that the most important features are not so much the disease processes involved but the original personality of the patient, the amount of function possible and the society and situation in which she, or he, lives.

That the return of physical function is not always in direct proportion with the degree of recovery from the original disease process is well illustrated by the strange natural history of *MRS. STOWICK.*

Some twelve years ago Mrs. Stowick was struck down by a left-sided stroke whilst she was at her place of work in central London. Consequently she was taken to the nearest hospital. She was treated intensively for two weeks and failed to make progress, and so she was moved to the less pressed country branch of the hospital—many miles from her own home. There, the vigorous process of rehabilitation was carried on, with no apparent return of capability, and after about six or eight weeks of this unrewarding treatment, Mrs. Stowick (still only in her late fifties) was shipped off to the geriatric hospital nearest to her home. She was there abandoned to a bedfast existence in a very crowded ward. She had, in the well-known parlance, "been disposed of".

A potent factor in the failure to remobilise Mrs. Stowick may have been related to her difficult home life. She had been the breadwinner and family support as her husband was an unemployed alcoholic. The relief in laying down long sustained burdens and herself becoming the recipient of care must have been considerable. Her motivation towards personal independence, coupled with the prospect of resumption of her responsibilities, was understandably minimal. Her one child was married and geographically well removed from the situation.

Four years later her husband died. By this time the home had gone and her situation was not conducive to renewed efforts towards rehabilitation. She was well and truly marooned amongst the 'chronic sick' and permanent hospital residents.

By chance, her child and family moved into our area, and after some years of commuting across London week in and week out to visit Mrs. Stowick, they prevailed upon the hospitals concerned to arrange a transfer.

Mrs. Stowick then arrived amongst us, after twelve years of lying almost flat in a hospital cot-sided bed. Mentally, she was very alert and orientated, and she had retained an intact and lively personality by continuous book and newspaper reading. Her speech was a little slurred as she was not used to conversing very much. Physically, she was obese and inert.

In the natural course of events, she was sat out of bed the day after her arrival, and her spine-chilling screams brought staff running from all quarters. When the hullabaloo subsided and coherence was re-established, she explained that the 'vast' area of open floor confronting her, when she was sitting in a chair looking across the ward, had terrified her. It had made her sick and dizzy. (We have always considered our wards overcrowded and were dumbfounded!) She had been accustomed to bed occupancy of a ward of closely packed beds—four rows, the centre ones back to back, with only room for a small locker between the beds and a narrow passage-way between the foot ends. Having lain in one place for almost twelve years, the sudden change of position and space had completely unnerved her.

For many weeks we had to maintain her in one of the old-fashioned, high-sided cot beds, at her own insistence. Gradually she was weaned to a low bed with small telescopic rails which she finds useful to pull on when turning a little in bed or helping to sit up. She sits out in a chair for increasing periods of time. From there she will progress to a wheel-chair, one hopes a self-propelled, one-armed drive chair. She will join the others in the work groups and for dining. New clothes may be a further exciting incentive to a woman who previously took interest in her appearance; a new hair-do goes without saying.

Her family live close to the hospital and they have numerous friends, which means that she has many more visitors. If all goes according to plan, she should soon be able to leave the confines of hospital and go and visit her family at home.

For our part, we must give her security and support and we must guarantee her a sheltered environment for as long as she has need. If she has adequate confidence in our integrity in this respect, then there is little doubt, even at this belated stage, that she will return to personal independence. The door can never and should never be closed.

> "Life can only be understood backwards—
> but it must be lived forwards."
>
> *Søren Kierkagaard*

References

1. Binks, F. Allen. (1968). *Brit. Med. J.*, **i**, 269-74.
2. Ritchie, Douglas. (1960). *"Stroke. A Diary of Recovery". London. Faber & Faber, Ltd.* Pp. 174. *Price* 12*s*. 6*d*.
3. Ritchie, Evelyn. Personal Communication.

Chapter Two

RELATIVES' CONFERENCE

"Hospitals are essentially artificial establishments, inevitably orientated to the sick and inevitably outside normal society to a great degree. There are no places for those whose need is for normal or very near normal society".[1]

Mention was made earlier of the fact that of every five visits made to people at home, on an average only on two occasions is admission to hospital found to be the appropriate recommendation. Basically, in five times out of five, admission to hospital has been explicitly underlying the original request for help or advice from the referring family doctor.

What then happens to the residual three? Sometimes there is a need for an almost ludicrously simply piece of advice, or provision of an aid. The most satisfying examples of this were far from infrequent a few years ago; one could almost diagnose the pattern and the need on reading the doctor's referral. The story would read roughly as follows: "Mrs. Smith was discharged from X hospital ten days ago—she had been admitted there several weeks ago following a fall which caused a fractured neck of femur. She returned home, ambulant, but is now bedfast and helpless. She cannot be managed at home."

A visit to Mrs. Smith would find an apprehensive, demoralised lady, lying in bed, with either an exhausted, resentful family or anxious neighbours standing by, saying, "She should never have been sent home like that". Always, reposing dustily in some corner, one would find an elegant pair of crutches, mutely telling the experienced observer the unhappy story.

The story is one of application of skill and techniques to a technical problem, without thought of the person or the person's

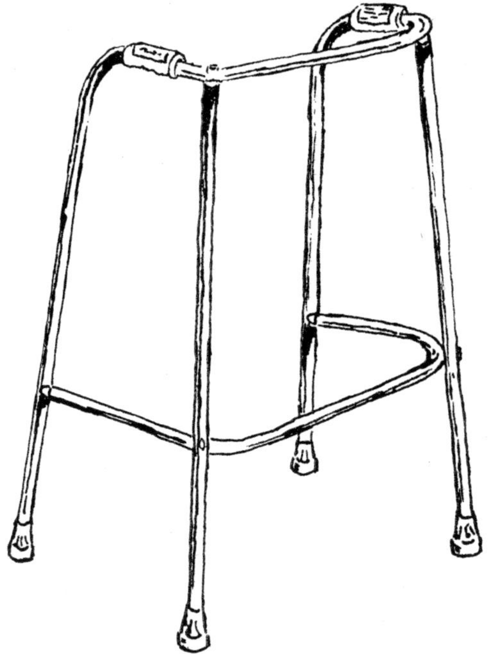

Figure 6. *Walking Frame*

need in his own environment. In other words, the fractured femur had been pinned and plated expertly by the surgeons and the physiotherapists had taken over. The patient had been remobilised, had probably graduated from walking between parallel bars to crutch-walking, had gone up and down the steps in the department (with hand-rails on either side), had proved her ability to do everything for herself and had then been discharged home—a perfect result.

Unfortunately, there are all sorts of hazards at home—stairs much steeper—no adequate hand-rails—steps to the lavatory—beds with sagging frames and of the wrong height. Crutches, too, have a habit of falling; one cannot put them down easily while attending to chores, and carrying objects whilst using them is incredibly difficult. The answer to all these problems could usually be provided on the spot by explanation, demonstration of the patient's function and capability to family and neighbours and provision of a four-legged walking aid, such as a walking frame (*Figure* 6—*see page* 29). These frames remain where they are stood, can be leant on with one hand whilst the other is in use and generally give the patient much more feeling of security, support and confidence. Commonsense adaptation to furniture, such as making a firm base for the bed, with boards across the frame under mattress, placing a commode of appropriate height by the bed for night use, and removal of dangerous mats, are all easy manoeuvres, but the amount of improvement in morale and confidence they produce is out of all proportion to the effort involved.

If one goes about one's visits endeavouring to understand the needs of the people visited and also being only too aware of the limited resources of space and staff behind one, a new dimension begins to emerge in one's work. "Traditional problems are often the result of traditional ways of acting and thinking",[2] is indeed only too true. Where there is a high proportion of hospital beds available in comparison with the population at risk, one finds that too often the method used for solving personal difficulties in a home is hospital admission. Small wonder that resolution of the problems rarely occurs, and after a time the patient is discharged home, with nothing changed, and sooner or later breaks again on the self-same rocks.

This matter of communication with relatives and friends came home to us very clearly in 1961. Mr. and Mrs. Douglas Ritchie spelt out to us very forcibly the needs of the supporting relative for information and positive help in learning how best to assist a disabled person. In our Geriatric Unit we prided ourselves on team-work—the visiting of a patient at home before admission —the planning of his programme to fit in with his needs and functions—the close communication between all concerned with this programme, including the patient. Somehow, however, we seemed to have given very little thought to the key figure in all these negotiations—that is, the supporting relative or friend. We knew that, contrary to press, radio, Ministerial and official opinion, many relatives were all too responsible,[5] conscientious and duty-motivated. In fact, we often remarked that it was the patient treated with too much solicitude who was the greater problem, rather than the one who had been callously neglected, for the latter retained more personal independence, whilst the former had had it sapped and drained away by over-protection and smothering solicitude.

This meeting with Mr. and Mrs. Ritchie caused us to review our methods. It seemed as though we were treating the body fairly effectively but we were only paying lip-service to the mind. We had not been following our reasoning through, for once personal independence is regained, there must be incentive and support to maintain it outside hospital. People need the stimulus of other people and of needful things to do. Creature comforts and the sight of familiar faces and things around one are not sufficient stimulus to live life to the full. Relatives at home need this explained to them or else they feel guilt and remorse at their inability to maintain the apparent miraculous cure that the hospital team often produces with their professional competence and expertise. Relatives obviously needed all the information and explanation or help we could give them in order to understand the situation in which they found themselves.

In September, 1961, we launched a new venture to try and help bridge this gap between hospital and home. We arranged to have a regular evening meeting on the last Thursday of every month. We called it the Relatives' Discussion Group—later Relatives' Conference[3]—and tentatively and timorously we proceeded to learn an enormous amount about management, incentive and patients' and relatives' reactions—to their problems, to each other, to the hospital and to officialdom in general. It is a frightening thing to well-protected hospital staff to be exposed suddenly to the public at large, with no holds barred! We had expected initially to have only one-way communication—'us' to 'them'—and we started off with neat little demonstrations of how things should be done, i.e. how beds should be made—dressing problems tackled—the 'right' way for a stroke patient to get up from a chair or come downstairs.

The public was polite—listened, and gradually, with the utmost kindness, they began to educate us as to how life is really lived; how difficulties are actually coped with and overcome.

Instead of using lithe students as models for demonstrations, the patients themselves came to the meetings, and together, patient and relative would demonstrate their difficulties. Sometimes the experts would help towards a solution; sometimes some other member of the meeting would offer a solution they had worked out. There was one glorious evening, when much solemn thought had been given to the problem of getting a very heavy, arthritic stroke lady from a lying position to a sitting position in bed. She was at that stage an in-patient in hospital and it was always necessary to have two members of staff to do this. The physiotherapist tried all known techniques for single-handed action recommended for this situation, and failed. How then was the patient's daughter to manage at home—an elderly lady herself with a known bad heart and a not very strong back? During all these manoeuvres the daughter had sat silent and observant and on being invited directly to join in, she came forward and demonstrated how she actually did manage each morning, single handed, to get her mother from a lying to a sitting position in bed; she used, as a sort of lever, her exceedingly protuberant and pendulous abdomen! It was collapse of the thin not the stout party, as Mr. Punch might have remarked.

One wonders why experts in hospital (and other places) are so reluctant to admit bafflement. Why are we so frightened of two-way communication? One remembers the very disabled man with multiple sclerosis, being supported single handed at home by a devoted wife. This man was incapable of doing anything for himself except actually chewing his own food. He was a clear call on hospital support if ever there was one, but his wife wished to look after him at home and she had evolved a workable regime and timetable for managing at home. Like everyone, however, she felt the need of a holiday once a year, and at first, attempts were made to give the husband a holiday too, but this proved unsuccessful. Each time the wife had been sent for to take him home because he was disrupting the establishment in which he was staying, particularly at night. This meant that she had to give up going on holiday or else accept hospitality for him from the local hospital during the relevant period; this, both husband and wife had been reluctant to do. Our help was sought and a minute record made of the man's routine so that this could be continued in hospital. Unhappily, one factor was overlooked—or rather the implications were not fully realised. Lying in one position for more than two hours at night produced great pain and consequently the wife was accustomed to wake up and turn the patient over. If this was not done, he became distressed and created considerable noise and disturbance which, at home, brought complaints from the neighbours. Instructions were given to the night staff to do the turning, and all should have been well. Unfortunately, it was found that it required three nurses in order to turn the patient and the ward had only two nurses on duty at night and a third could not always be found in time, two-hourly. Consequently, pandemonium reigned over the week-end and when sister came back on duty on the Monday, she found a very sorry situation indeed. She quickly telephoned the wife for help and got her to come and demonstrate to the staff her method for turning the patient single handed.

This story should have had a happy ending but unfortunately it had not, for the two traumatic days took their toll, plus the effects of the heavier night sedation necessary, in order to give the patient relief and other patients sleep when regular turning had not been possible. Pressure sores had developed; the patient had to be kept in bed in order to heal the sores; his morale dropped; he developed bronchopneumonia, and as so often happens in a hospital ward, this was caused by a particularly virulent and resistant organism. The patient died, leaving a wife consumed with resentment and distress and a hospital staff similarly upset. And yet at no point had there been anything but goodwill and a tremendous desire to help husband and wife retain their independence.

One could say with hindsight—if only we had asked the wife not only to stay at home for the first week of admission, before going away for her holiday, in case anything went wrong, but also to come into the hospital and instruct us in her methods of coping, so that there would have been a smooth hand-over. It seems such a patently sensible thing to do but it is only as I actually write down this poignant incident that the obvious, the glaring defect, strikes me. Our communication cannot be really and truly two-way until we, the hospital team, are just as willing to *be shown how*, as we are to go out of hospital into the home *to demonstrate*.

That our Relatives' Conference opened up the channel of communication, there could be no doubt. In the early days we had two incidents of relatives who came to the meetings month after month, which was an unexpected and unusual pattern. The patients concerned had both been seen on domiciliary visits and neither had needed hospital admission, chiefly because of the devoted ministrations of the two daughters involved, giving full-time support. Both daughters, however, had needed reassurance that they were doing as much, if not more, than the experts.

The first daughter had been unaware that we had been approached by the family doctor. She had been caring for her father in bed for two years with the aid of her husband and son and the district nurse. She had only been to the doctor's surgery to obtain a prescription for a supply of dressings. Whether the district nurse had suggested to the doctor that hospital was required we shall never know, for it transpired that he himself had not visited the household for at least six months. When the hospital physician arrived on the doorstep, the daughter was extremely incensed and belligerent and it took a considerable amount of time and persuasion, firstly to be invited into the house and secondly to be allowed to see and examine the patient. Once her confidence was won, anxieties and worries as to whether she was doing the right thing, etc., poured out. But it was patently obvious that the patient was enjoying, and was completely fixed in, his role and admission to hospital would have done more harm than good, so reassurance was possible. Daughter and son-in-law came to three or four monthly meetings, asked all the questions they had been storing up, came again for a refresher evening six months later to ask help with a fresh query and then were seen no more. There was a sequel—a letter eighteen months later to say that the father had died peacefully at home where they and he wished him to be and to die, and that the daughter and son-in-law were extremely grateful for all the help and support they had received from us.

The other case was different—this was a widower father and unmarried daughter of some 50-odd years, living together. Father had had a mild stroke—the daughter welcomed the home visit of the hospital physician, and as the latter happened to be a woman, felt freer to express some of her problems, a number of which related to the natural constraints a sheltered spinsterhood had imposed on her. Her ignorance of male anatomy could have been the subject of great ribaldry under any other circumstances. The main problem, once the question of hospital or not had been resolved, was whom to have to blanket bath the patient. The very kind and good neighbour next door was a trained nurse, and had offered, but the old man felt modestly that he would be shy when in future they chatted over the garden fence. We decided that the impersonal district nurse was the most obvious and circumspect choice, and she was duly invited. It was some time before I heard the sequel to this. The old man was a very keen Old Time dancing enthusiast and the district nurse, when she arrived, turned out to be one of his favourite dancing partners!

The daughter gladly accepted our invitation to the Relatives' Conference and arranged for someone to sit with her father the evenings she came. She was a fascinated and vociferous participant in the proceedings; she came early and was the last to go. When she came the following month and five subsequent times, we became worried. Was this her only escape? Did she only feel free to leave the old man when it was a question of attending hospital? Should we tackle her on this? Possibly the most disconcerting feature of her visits was her rapt attention to the film on stroke rehabilitation we showed (at that time, "New Beginnings"[4]). She sat through it, completely absorbed and attentive. In the meantime her father had been up to the Out-Patient Clinic and attended occupational therapy for assessment and had been discharged from all attendance, completely independent again. Then her visits stopped abruptly—we felt lost and anxiously checked with one another but no one had said anything unkind. It was inexplicable. Later that year, at the end of one summer month, she came again—not to the film but to the discussion part of the evening, and at an appropriate moment, shyly told the assembled company how much attending the meetings had helped her; how she had watched the film each month and had seen something new at each showing. When she felt more confident in her own capabilities, she had stopped coming. Then one day her father had fallen whilst out in the garden. She panicked momentarily and then remembered having seen the physiotherapist demonstrate various ways of helping disabled people to get up from the ground. She made her father comfortable whilst she recollected what to do next and was full of joy when she found the method worked.

It was some years later that I heard in a casual conversation with the family doctor that this fine old man had continued to lead a very active life—even returning to his Old Time dancing—and had died suddenly and swiftly one day, metaphorically with his boots on and in full vigour. This to us seems the acme of a success story—to support people and enable them to find their own solutions and work out their own best methods of achieving independence.

"In my beginning is my end".
T. S. Eliot

References

1. Binks, F. Allen. (1962). *Lancet,* **i,** 1083-86.
2. *Ibidem.* (1964). **ii,** 1233-36.
3. Hawker, M. B. (1964). *Lancet,* **i,** 1098.
4. "*New Beginnings*"—Film on Stroke Rehabilitation. Produced by Geriatric Unit, Bromley Group Hospital Management Committee, 1960.
5. Townsend, P. et al. (1968). *Old People in Three Industrial Societies.* Routledge and Kegan Paul. Page 478 ,"In Denmark 20 per cent pensionable population live with children; in USA, 27 per cent; in UK, 42 per cent."

Chapter Three

FURTHER ACTIVITY CENTRE

"A practical physician must consider the personal as well as the impersonal. He must use the correct tools for the problems he encounters. It is futile to try to uncork a bottle with a tin opener".[1]

Open session discussion at the Relatives' Conference helped with general information and explanation and even with some specific problems; but before long it became apparent that many individual and personal problems needed a more limited gathering of people, with peace and privacy in which to work things out.

This posed a problem in itself as space is always a vital question with us. There are no Day Rooms on our wards in the main hospital and the formal physiotherapy and occupational therapy departments are crowded most of the day. Where then could we find peace and privacy? It took eighteen months of endeavour, cajolery and administrative strategy before we managed to have the lean-to corrugated shed attached to the Unit offices, lined, linoed and repaired as a waiting room with an adjoining small room, similarly lined, carpeted and fitted with a hand-rail along one wall. At the same time a lavatory was built in the waiting room. There was little room for therapeutic equipment but we were, in fact, not anxious to have much, as we wished the surroundings to be as home like as possible. Further, there were three broad steps leading from the shed into our main office, and with the aid of the hospital plumber, a very strong gas piping rail was put up the centre of these steps, with a stout vertical post at the top. This provided excellent practice steps for either right or left hemiplegic patients—plus a turn at the top.

Having achieved our room, with carpet, low bed, commode and several different kinds and heights of armchair, we were complete. All we lacked was a name for the place. Lean-To-Shed seemed depressing; Out-Patient Clinic too pompous; Functional Assessment Unit might give the wrong connotation to our professional brethren. Eventually we called it the Further Activity Centre—a rather nice play on words being intended here, as we were implying the need not so much for further activity on the part of the patient, but more the need for further activity on the part of the professional. (A Re-Think Place was a discarded suggestion!).

To anyone who is not steeped in medical training and hospital traditions, it would seem the most obvious thing in the world that, if one is dealing with an adult person with many facets and many problems, the reasonable thing to do would be to gather together a collection of experts who might be able to help. Then a concerted effort can be made with the experts, the patient and those mainly concerned with him at home, to talk about the problems and try to work out the solutions. Time spent in this fashion might save months of isolated effort. The traditional method for dealing with a patient's difficulties is to send the patient from department to department to have the various components of his particular disability dealt with by the various experts in their various departments, and often there is very little communication or connection between these experts. Consequently, one can have the makings of a Whitehall farce. The patient who goes down to physiotherapy to have walking exercises, but who returns to the ward and expects the nurse to push him to the lavatory in a wheel-chair, is an example: he looks on walking as exercise treatment and not related to the functions of everyday living, and considers that he's had his daily dose of treatment, thank you.

Or there is the man who has been assessed in the Functional Assessment Unit and found to be able to dress himself perfectly competently, but who may be dressed and undressed each day by the extremely busy nurse who is trying to get 15 or 20 patients up or back to bed, single handed, and who has no time to stand back and allow the patient to do things slowly for himself.

This, of course, is not just a problem of hospital life; I recall very vividly, visiting a family who were bombarding their family doctor to take action and have them relieved of the intolerable burden of the wife's old aunt who had worn them all out. It was an incredible story of a rather unspontaneous, passive maiden lady of 85 who had always lived with a dominant elder sister in the Midlands. The dominant old lady had died; the younger one had deteriorated and neglected herself and when the cold weather came she took to her bed, in a very poor state, being found helpless there by neighbours and whisked off to hospital. In time, the niece in London was located, a discharge notice issued and the old lady delivered to the niece's door in an ambulance, before she had time to think. Having travelled south, firstly by ambulance from hospital to train and then from the London station to the niece's home by ambulance, she was cold, frightened and exhausted on arrival and was carried into the house by the kindly ambulance men. From then on, she had been the object of the most tremendous solicitude, the niece undressing and washing her and helping her in and out of bed, on and off the commode and in and out of a chair. When the niece's back had given out, her husband had taken over, even arranging his work so that he could rush home at midday to assist the patient on and off the commode.

When the hospital physician arrived post-haste, having been persuaded by the family doctor that this was a matter of utmost urgency, requiring immediate hospital admission, the husband and wife were at breaking point. It was, by then, the end of the summer, and they were nearing their long-booked and long anticipated annual holiday. Their own daughter, an ex-nurse, had offered to come and stay in the house and look after the old lady. The daughter already had two small children and another on the way—how could she possibly cope with all the work entailed? The problem indeed sounded grim, and having found out as much background detail as possible, the visiting physician was astounded to walk into the next room and find a charming looking, very rosy, healthy and beautifully groomed old lady sitting cosily in an armchair, shelling peas. Her main handicap was a considerable impairment of hearing. She gave her version of her illness, having few complaints apart from rheumatism, and on brief physical examination was found to have normal power and practically full range of movement in all her limbs.

Somewhat puzzled, the doctor invited her to get up and

walk a little. The niece rushed forward to assist, offering to get her husband in to help too but, with some difficulty, was dissuaded from either course. The old lady rose, unaided, from her chair and, holding on to the back of a handy wooden bedroom chair to steady herself, walked happily across the room. The niece dissolved into hysteria, screamed for her husband and hurled abuse at the old lady. She was taken away to an adjoining room to be comforted by the husband and when she was calmer, the husband left her, to accompany the doctor into the patient's room to witness this miracle. Again the old lady got up, walked across the room, demonstrated her ability to get on and off the bed and, as a *tour de force,* went up and down some stairs. The husband was dumbfounded. "Why", he demanded, "had you never done this for us?" The old lady replied simply, "You have never asked me to." She had acquiesced in their attentions, thought it odd the way they had waited on her hand and foot, but had come to the conclusion that they liked doing it and had thought it best to humour them as they were being kind enough to give her a home.

This story does not end there, for once more truth is proved to be even more unbelievable than fiction. This hurried visit had been paid in the morning because in the afternoon the Geriatric Department was having a 'demonstration' meeting of the Relatives' Conference in honour of a party of occupational therapists attending their International Congress, which was being held in London. We had invited to our meeting the area welfare officer of a local borough (then part of Middlesex County Council) to speak about his work. He related to us some of the pressures and problems, and how that very morning he had to try and find an emergency vacancy somewhere in one of the Middlesex Welfare Homes for a lady who did not even belong to the area but who had recently been transferred from the Midlands. He had at last managed to secure a vacancy at a designated Home a long way away and he did not relish having to do this sort of thing in this way. Slowly, the pieces fitted together and it became clear that under the pressure of the relatives' importunings, the family doctor had approached both statutory authorities—the welfare and the hospital service—for help and both had responded with alarming alacrity. The only difference was that the doctor from the hospital had been able to examine the patient and try her out whilst the welfare officer had had to accept the position as presented to him. Fortunately it was possible for the two departments to co-operate. The hospital admitted the patient for a very short spell indeed, in order to make sure that the patient was confident of her own abilities, and then she went to one of the smaller residential homes near to her niece.

If, at that time, our Further Activity Centre had been available, there would have been no need to use the rather cumbersome apparatus of hospital admission to re-establish everyone's confidence in the patient's capabilities. This, indeed, was trying to uncork a bottle with a tin opener!

Sentimentally, one would have wished for a marvellous reconciliation between aunt and niece and family and her return to them to live happily ever after. But this is not how life is lived. The whole history of this affair was doomed to failure from square one. If there had been any family closeness in the first place, the patient would never have got into the state she did, which landed her in hospital in the Midlands. Imperative discharge to next of kin without a by-your-leave is rarely successful in promoting happy relationships, and the paucity of information accompanying the patient, plus the absence of medical support this end, made disaster almost inevitable. The wonder is that any sort of relationship was preserved at all. The niece visited her aunt regularly and also had her home at intervals. The marvel is that she was able to overcome her mixed feelings of resentment and guilt sufficiently to do this.

Here is a wonderful occasion for society to point the finger and say scornfully, "Irresponsible relatives trying to off-load their responsibilities on to the State". But when one looks more into the pattern of the whole incident, cannot one say, "over-conscientious relatives?" If they had exercised their prerogative and point blank refused responsibility in the first place, the patient would have had to remain in the Midland hospital, and arrangements would have had to be made for placement in a residential Home locally. At least this would have kept the patient in an area she knew, where she was presumably known and where she might even have had some acquaintances. As it is, she is a stranger to her present area, with only her niece and family to maintain her contacts with the outside world.

Dr. John Smith gave the summary to this incident in 1666—"The reasons why persons in this Age fall so soon into this decrepit state and why the miseries thereof are so multiplied and magnified on them is because either they call not soon enough for help or because those that are called in either understood not or minde not what they aught to do. An honest and able physician may surely approve himself to this ancient patient, a restorer of life, a nourisher of old age".

Having digressed yet again, let us return to the Further Activity Centre (FAC) and its function. It is difficult to describe how subtly it has become an integral part in the department's way of life. At first we found it a great boon for our out-patient use, but here we met the hazard of ambulance transport which is very erratic and irregular; as our staff are all part time, it meant much time being wasted, waiting for patients to arrive. Our wards were a quarter of a mile away across the hospital grounds, so that it was not easy to do other things whilst awaiting ambulance arrivals. Again, it was necessary to rely on internal hospital transport to bring in-patients over. Ultimately we came to the conclusion that the best method of transport for out-patients, if relatives had no car of their own, was for a car-owning member of the team to go out and bring the patient in from home (sometimes a kindly district nurse or health visitor would do this). For in-patients, one of the team would push them through the hospital grounds, and therefore one was very much at the mercy of the weather! It is interesting how many excellent schemes fail through the vagaries, or sheer lack, of transport.

Recently the whole department headquarters has been moved to a hutted settlement close to the medical wards—something we have wanted for many years. This is a vast improvement but still by no means perfect, for our wards are at the top of the building and there is only one passenger and service lift and still an open-air walk or ride of fifty yards before reaching our building. Once there, however, things are much better; the carpeted room is bigger, and opening off it is a small functional kitchen which is very helpful occupational therapy-wise.

In parenthesis, this new accommodation is also very helpful for our Relatives' Conferences. Previously we had to show our film in one place and then transfer to the Occupational Therapy Department to have the rest of the meeting, with a break in between for relatives to visit the wards at the scheduled visiting time. This made a very broken and long evening, but despite this, it has been a flourishing concern for over six years.

Since our move, we have felt it possible to have a change of form—long overdue some of us feel. This is even more possible with the new extended visiting hours on the wards. For a long time the Relatives' Conference has been more of a do-it-yourself event with only three fixed items—film, tape-recording and coffee, but now we are leaving the arrangements more and more to interested relatives. They are starting off by organising refreshments, aided by a local youth group which has expressed interest in "doing welfare work with old people". The hospital team will always be available but more as a part of the community discussion than as actual leaders or initiators. For the first of the new sessions we invited the original paid organiser of Voluntary Workers for the Fulbourn Hospital pilot scheme, Mrs. Chrystal King, to tell us her experiences[2]. It was a tremendous success and with an audience of 50 avid pairs of ears, a small nucleus of interested people was found. So it seems more than likely that our Further Activity Centre can also become a focal *social activity centre* for our patients and their relatives in the way that T. D. Hunter advocated, as long ago as 1963, in the *Lancet*[3]: "instead of being a mere 'supporting' service, the hospital must concentrate on becoming the dynamic centre of the socio-medical services and the active sponsor of preventive health in the community."

Having a larger area of room for our FAC has enabled us to enlarge the scope of our regular fortnightly staff meeting which is held early in the morning. It can now be thrown open to our colleagues in the three neighbouring Health and Welfare Departments and we can invite local family doctors as well. We have found in the past that if a meeting is known to be held regularly and an open invitation offered, people seem much more likely to drop in as and when they can, and at times of particular need.

The art of communication in these compartmentalised days

is long and difficult. Providing a regular channel of informal communication, and ensuring that the lines are kept open, is even more difficult. Our efforts only seem the merest drops in the great sea of need but at least, if some breaches are made in the high hospital walls and the outside world tramps in and out through them often enough, the rest of the earthworks will soon crumble and perhaps in a few years' time there will not be even a line of demarcation to be seen betwixt hospital and the community.

This is all very fine and pie-in-the-sky, my reader will be saying—especially the hospital worker who feels beset, beleaguered and rushed off his feet. It must be nice to work at Edgware and have all these social jamborees, but when do they see and treat patients? This FAC was designed to help sick elderly people. Who is doing the *real* work? Let us then pass swiftly on to contemplate one of the first patients 'treated' in the FAC.

MRS. DRESDEN, a 76-year-old lady, first came to our notice in October. A domiciliary visit was requested for advice as to whether a wheel-chair or walking frame would be the most useful aid; she was too frail to attend the Out-Patient Clinic.

A visit was paid first on the morning of the last Thursday in October—a significant date, as will be apparent later. This lady's history was as follows:

Mrs. Dresden normally lived on the other side of London with her very crippled 78-year-old husband, who had such severe osteo-arthritis of his hips that he had to live on the ground floor of their house, being unable to climb stairs. She slept upstairs and when one night six weeks previously he heard a crash on the floor above, he had to find a neighbour to come and see what had happened. Mrs. Dresden had had a stroke affecting her left side. At first their only child, Mrs. Love, stayed with them. She then visited daily from her own home in Edgware until eventually, when Mrs. Dresden was fit enough, they bundled her into the son-in-law's car and brought her back to stay with them. Mr. Dresden remained at home, supported by a home help once a week and meals-on-wheels twice a week, the other midday meals being sent across from a café opposite. The daughter visited at the week-end to supplement the services and a district nurse called in once a week also.

On Mrs. Dresden's arrival at her daughter's house, she was tenderly installed in the best bedroom; a commode and cantilever table and backrest were obtained and she was cherished in a way that defies description. Perhaps the fact that Mrs. Love was a second wife, and her husband had a grown-up son and she herself had no children may have had some bearing on the situation.

The visiting hospital physician found Mrs. Dresden sitting in an armchair close to her bed, packed round with cushions and muffled in rugs in a spotless and warm room with radio to hand and a view on to the garden for visual solace. The doctor's comment at the time was that she probably had to swallow her own food but there was very little else she was allowed to do for herself. She was not dressed. She could walk with help. The family doctor had forbidden stairs more than once a day and consequently she only went downstairs in the evening, when Mr. Love came home from work. The stairs were steep and had a treacherous twist at the top, and one could see that they would present difficulties for her.

It was suggested gently to the daughter that she should let Mrs. Dresden live more dangerously and adventurously—that she would regain independence much more quickly if she were allowed to do more for herself—but the words fell on deaf ears. Six weeks of giving the uttermost in tender loving care seemed to have dulled Mrs. Love's perceptive powers; so it seemed some dramatic and heroic effort would be needed to break into this strangling circle of solicitude. In the meantime Mrs. Dresden looked pleadingly at the doctor, for she had whispered in a moment when the daughter was absent answering the telephone, that she felt she could do more but did not want to upset her daughter who had been so good to her.

This seemed the sort of situation for which the Further Activity Centre was ideally suited, but unfortunately this was still during the eighteen month struggle to obtain the Centre and it was by no means ready. Then the date was recollected, and after much discussion and persuasion it was arranged that the daughter and mother should attend the Relatives' Conference that evening. The fortunate snag then appeared: there would be no chance to warn Mr. Love, and Mrs. Love would therefore have to remain at home to give him his meal and explain the circumstances, after which they could then both come on to the hospital. Meanwhile the physician would call and take Mrs. Dresden to the meeting on her own. This proved an ideal arrangement, though, as Mrs. Love helped get her mother into the car, she was almost distraught with anxiety. Mrs. Dresden, however, was like a child released from school, and once she had thrown off the infective tensions from the household, she chatted very freely about her problems.

At the meeting that evening there were several very much more disabled people and their relatives, and on hearing some of Mrs. Dresden and Mrs. Love's story they offered advice from their own experience, and so the ice cracked. Mr. Love proved to be an old TB patient with a tremendous amount of hospital experience who came initially at the end of the meeting to take his wife and mother-in-law home, but he was so impressed by the informality that he came to the whole meeting the following two months, just to see if the atmosphere was genuine. (He commented on how things change, recalling his own experiences in the sanatorium days and the once weekly weighing ritual: he had never been allowed to stand facing the weights, and when he had asked what his weight was he had been told off very roundly and instructed to mind his own business!).

By coming to the Out-Patient Clinic and sessions at the Occupational Therapy Department, we gradually cut a few threads of Mrs. Dresden's silver cord, until such time as the Further Activity Centre was at last watertight and reasonably warm. Then we were able to gather together with mother and daughter and really demonstrate how capable Mrs. Dresden was, at the same time giving our medical social worker a chance to open up the question of the future in more open session. Up until then, it was assumed by Mrs. Love that her mother would take up permanent residence with the Love's and Mr. Dresden stay where he was. There seemed to have been no discussion on this, but we knew it was not what Mrs. Dresden had in her mind as she had voiced her desire to return to her own home as fast as possible, despite the onset of winter.

Soon Mrs. Dresden was being allowed to attend the hospital out-patients on her own (before the daughter had always accompanied her and waited) and then we felt the time had come for Mrs. Dresden to venture further afield. By a series of complex arrangements (transport difficulties again), Mrs. Dresden was taken on the strength of the local Elderly People's Workrooms, three days a week. This was early in January. She worked two hours in the workrooms in the afternoons and drew her 1s. 3d. per hour with her fellow-workers. More strands of the cord were severed.

Gradually, with everyone pulling in the same direction and with communication going between our medical social worker and the health visitor in Mr. Dresden's area, plans were forming. The Dresden's would sell their house and if a suitable bungalow or flat could be found near the Love's, they would both move in. Then disaster struck. Mr. Dresden fell on the ice in the back garden and lay helpless until a neighbour found him. He tried to manage at home for a week but it became too much and he was admitted to his local geriatric hospital.

Meanwhile the Loves went ahead searching for accommodation and arranging for the sale of the old home. The sale went through before arrangements were made for the new accommodation, and here a rather sad note creeps into the tale. Mr. Dresden was, and is, a greatly handicapped man, with very severe osteo-arthritis of his hips and knees, completely unable to bend down or do steps of any kind. He had also developed severe deep ulcerations on his legs during his stay in hospital and it had been accepted that he could not manage alone, nor had the daughter room in her small house to put up a bed for him downstairs. Consequently, he had been unwillingly accepted in hospital until such time as alternative accommodation was ready. Unwillingly, one surmises, for as soon as the sale of the house was through, arrangements were made by the other hospital to transfer the patient, willy-nilly, to a nursing home in this area. In vain the daughter and son-in-law protested that it was going to take all the capital available to purchase a flat for Mr. and Mrs. Dresden and the very heavy fees of the nursing home would make tremendous inroads into the slender sum. They were told that Mr. Dresden was blocking a bed and that as he now had money (surely a *non sequitur,* when one considers need rather than finance), he must use it on a nursing home. When one considers that the more reasonable nursing homes in the area charge anything between 18-24 guineas a week, one can appreciate the family's dilemma. Protests were over-ridden (the family too responsible and conscientious to use their prerogative and refuse to be coerced in this manner) and Mr. Dresden was duly transferred to a nursing home, with one day's warning.

Consequently, when the flat purchase was completed there was no money left for any new furnishings or luxuries, and the couple had to go to National Assistance for the first time in their lives.

"When sorrows come, they come not single spies but in battalions".

William Shakespeare

References

1. Binks, F. Allen. (1964). *Lancet,* **ii,** 1233-36.
2. Clark, D. H., & King, E.M.C. (1966). *Lancet,* **i,** 1088-90.
3. Hunter, T. D. (1963). *Lancet,* **ii,** 933-35.

Chapter Four

CUSTODIAL CARE

"Nobody seems to think of the disabled person as a person with a person's needs but rather as an object to be cared for".[1]

When Mrs. Dresden was firmly established at the Work Centre she attended the follow-up clinic infrequently and more for moral support than for medical treatment. Here one must face the difficulties inherent in running any attempt at personal service when the demands and pressures on that service from without are so great. Continuity of personnel is essential if one is hoping to identify need and provide help and support at the time it is required. Looking back now on this particular tangled skein of threads, one can see it as of "mingled yarn—good and ill together" and unhappily all the good strands are not emanating from our corner of the tangle and all the bad strands from some other corner. But this is the wretched hindsight again—one can see how things have happened and why they need not have happened in this way but one cannot say that they will not be allowed to happen thus again. Inevitably they will, because personnel are changing all the time and it is almost impossible to profit by each other's mistakes unless one is working as a member of a very tight-knit group, the persona of which is unvarying.

Our excuses are good; our alibis watertight; we have over one thousand requests for help each year and the number is steadily rising. Every one has to be sifted and dealt with in some way and the vast majority have to be gone into in some depth. How can the limited staff we have hope to tackle it all, in the way it should be done? In fact, how far should one go?

We are fortunate in that three of our doctors, one medical social worker, one occupational therapist and two secretaries have been constant members of the cast for at least seven years. But in this time we have had many house officers and locums, all extremely honourable, conscientious and valuable technical doctors but, with few exceptions, they have been birds of passage, travelling from the East to the West to pick up postgraduate experience and further diplomas before returning from whence they came. It is virtually impossible for them to hear what a patient is actually saying behind the facade of what a patient is and does. Therefore, examination and history taking can only be a technical exercise conducted on a scientific basis. The cultural undertones and lores must inevitably be lost. The only hope seems to lie in educating the consumer to make intelligible and obvious demands, when he has identified his own needs and has learnt to know what help is possible and available. This, perhaps, explains partially why, once having put our hand to the plough, in a sense, with Mrs. Dresden we should have somehow let it slip.

But it did, chiefly perhaps because Mrs. Dresden having had such responsible and devoted relatives who acquiesced in what they were told and were not vociferous in their demands for help, had made such a good recovery to personal independence. A ground floor maisonette was purchased and the old couple installed. The Welfare Department was approached for help, for, although it was a new ground floor maisonette with every modern convenience, there were three steep steps up to the front door and two steps out of the french windows into the garden, making Mr. Dresden more or less a prisoner. Unfortunately it was at that point that our help was virtually withdrawn and Mrs. Dresden was given an appointment to return for follow-up in one year's time. What was not known at this time was that the welfare officer had visited and had considered that the installation of a ramp would be expensive and would "only really complicate the situation".

Our next meeting with the family was another of those strange coincidences that seem more fictional than factual. The department was making a short film[2] of its activities to act as an illustration at an international meeting of *The Chest and Heart Association*. The subject was 'Stroke' and we remembered Mrs. Dresden as an excellent example of someone who had not only regained independence without having to be an in-patient in hospital, but who had also become an integrated member of a (to her) new community.

We telephoned Mrs. Dresden and Mrs. Love to explain things and ask if we could particularly film Mrs. Dresden at the Work Centre. Here was jolt one—she was no longer attending as it was too far by public transport and the son-in-law could not take her in his car. In fact, she was never leaving her maisonette at all except occasionally at week-ends when Mr. Love took her for a drive. Nevertheless, as time was so short, it was agreed to film her at the Centre and sort things out later. The doctor collected her from home and saw the flat and steep steps and met Mr. Dresden for the first time. It was then discovered that he still had considerable ulceration of his legs and the district nurse was having to visit daily and dress them. The constant exudate from the ulcers was a distress to everyone concerned. The doctor suggested to the daughter that she persuade the family doctor to refer Mr. Dresden to the Out-Patient Clinic as it seemed more than probable that the ulcers could be cleared up fairly quickly by the technique of weekly or two weekly application of impregnated dressings. Meanwhile, as Mrs. Dresden could not be transported to the Work Centre any more and as public transport around those parts was too erratic and dangerous, particularly in the cold weather, we had to think of some other means of getting Mrs. Dresden out of the house occasionally, independently of her family. The only available alternative was to bring her up by ambulance transport to a social Hospital Help Group that the Occupational Therapy Department had formed for the people who live in areas where there are no regular Work or Day Centres available. These people come up to the Occupational Therapy Department regularly, on one of two days a week, and help with the packing of dressings, etc., for the Central Sterile Supplies Department (CSSD). This tedious and monotonous work, much needed by the hospital, is enlivened by the animation of the two groups doing the work.

But still no word of Mr. Dresden's referral. It was not until three months later that Mrs. Love driven at last, not only to want help but also to make an effort to secure it (and driven, as so many dutiful, conscientious and responsible relatives are, by an impending holiday), came to the department's offices to ask for help and advice. In that time Mr. Dresden had got as far as attending the Dental Department, and was down on the surgeons' list to come in for a week and have his teeth removed and a minor surgical procedure done at the same time.

At last he was referred to the Geriatric Department, formally, and at last we could gather in a few more of the loose strands. Mr. and Mrs. Love were going on holiday in three months' time and taking Mrs. Dresden with them. Mr. Dresden would not be able to go, but on the other hand, they were not happy about leaving him alone in the house. Could he come into hospital for the relevant period?

It was explained that this would be no holiday for Mr. Dresden, nor did he have any need of hospital admission, but it would be a good idea for him to have a change of surroundings too. Had they thought of approaching the welfare authorities for help?

To cut a long story short, they did this, and a vacancy was found at one of the new Homes of the authority. Mr. Dresden, a very gregarious and friendly fellow, enjoyed it and was a popular guest. His legs had healed swiftly on the weekly dressing treatment, but they will always be at risk, as his peripheral circulation is so poor, and one visualises many difficulties before Mr. Dresden's span is o'er. He also comes to the CSSD Group, the alternate day from his wife, again purely a holding device until they can both attend the Work Centre when it is opened nearer to them. Here, of course, there will be much difficulty unless a ramp is built to the house and the Work Centre transport has a tail-lift hoist, for Mr. Dresden can only walk on the flat.

Two other interesting facets arose in these transactions, one of which was television. I mentioned previously that the financial resources of the Dresden's were swallowed up by the new flat, and as they had never had television and were virtually marooned indoors, Mr. and Mrs. Love gave them their older set and bought a new one for themselves. Came summer and all the sport programmes: Mrs. Love thought her father would be in clover, particularly as in his younger days he had frequently rowed at Henley. He looked forward to watching Henley with more enthusiasm even than a youngster has for Christmas. Came

Henley week, and it was only being transmitted on BBC2. The old set had not got BBC2. All became dust and ashes for Mrs. Love. Their new set had BBC 2 but she could not get her father to it, nor did she feel she could ask her husband to forego the new set after all he had already done for his in-laws. Furthermore, it would need a new aerial and he was already paying the licence, financing their telephone, etc. (Most people do not realise that for the normal housebound old person the telephone is completely beyond their means—a strange anomaly in this Welfare State. One would expect a telephone to be virtually a prescribable and necessary medical aid to the aged, frail, handicapped or housebound).

The other matter of interest was the ease with which well-known traps could be fallen into. The daughter mentioned to the doctor in passing at the Out-Patient Clinic that a wheel-chair would be of great value to her mother. They had recently taken her to the London Zoo and borrowed a wheel-chair there and pushed her round and she had enjoyed it very much. With a folding chair they could take her to Kew and other places and, better still, the daughter could take her to the local shops, letting Mrs. Dresden walk down the hill and pushing her back up if she was tired. When she realised these could be obtained fairly easily through the Ministry, she mentioned that when the ramp was in place, they would be able to take Mr. Dresden out in the car also and so two wheel-chairs were decided upon which could be folded and put in the boot of the car. Mr. Dresden was delighted at the thought of a wheel-chair and in due course measurements were taken, and the chairs ordered.

The chairs eventually came and all was expected to go merrily as a marriage bell. Not so. In the first place no one had consulted Mrs. Dresden and wild horses could not persuade her to submit to the ignominy of shopping in a wheel-chair. On her own feet or not at all would she go. Mr. Dresden was bitterly disappointed as he had anticipated a self-propelling chair in which he could get himself about the garden and street, apart from which, of course, no ramp had materialised and he was still a prisoner unless carried in and out of the house.

This situation is very much open-ended still. There will be several more chapters in this history before the case is closed, but it is a story that frightens me beyond measure. This is a family that has been known to be in difficulties for three years at least. They have asked for help on a number of occasions and have received some help. Many of their needs have been identified and spotlighted. Theoretically, no end of help can be given, yet in practice, how many of their needs have really been met by the community in which they live? Many agencies have come to know them, have made suggestions and taken desultory action, but who is actually co-ordinating any of these? Who is taking a personal interest to make sure that these things are happening—that their needs are being met? I would like to be able to say that at least our social workers are keeping their fingers on the pulse (there have been six different ones in the three years) and that our occupational therapists, physiotherapist or the doctor is holding a watching brief—at least a dozen hospital doctors have dealt with Mr. and Mrs. Dresden in this area alone. In the same way, numerous members of the Health and Welfare Departments of the Local Authority have been involved and one or two voluntary associations (we have tried to get a television set that has BBC 2 and also endeavoured to find voluntary visitors), but who has co-ordinated things? The only constant factors have been Mr. and Mrs. Dresden and Mr. and Mrs. Love and their family doctor.

Could he have been the co-ordinator of this vast and (to him) unseen army that he had somewhat unwittingly mustered? Theoretically, yes, he could have been. Factually, he would tell you he has not the time to do this, and I believe him. Would it have helped him, perhaps, if he had had a team attached to him? Supposing he had a health visitor and a district nurse specifically for his particular practice. Could one not visualise the possibility of more continuity, there on the spot where it was needed? Is this not precisely the place where there is a dire need of a co-ordinator and is not this just where the training and the experience of a health visitor is leading her? Just as in hospital, the doctor is useless without a nurse and a social worker to be his hands and eyes and ears, so surely is a family doctor equally handless, certainly, at any rate, in a busy suburban area. There is a great difference in small country areas where the whole population is virtually on one doctor's list and he therefore knows his patients very dimensionally indeed.

In discoursing on the unfinished saga of Mr. and Mrs. Dresden there occurs this question of holiday care. Have I mentioned how frequently we found that it is an impending holiday, that brings to the surface in a blaze, situations that may have been smouldering along unknown for months or more usually years?

One reads frequently in the medical press and elsewhere of hospitals that "ease the burden of hard-pressed relatives by taking their old people into hospital yearly (or even at more frequent intervals) in order to give the relatives a rest or a holiday". There are even some Geriatric Departments that have a slogan of "six weeks in and six weeks out". The workings of the human mind are indeed strange. When I first heard that slogan quoted some ten years ago and early in my 'geriatric' medical career, it used to fill me with suspicion and envy for a hospital that obviously must have a very high proportion of beds in relation to the population at risk, because I knew enough to realise, even then, that old people did not thrive on a roundabout system. I had already met many in my domiciliary visiting who had rotated at three or six monthly intervals round the homes of their various children. Always the circle had shrunk until the old person had ended up at the home of one of the children and goodwill had ultimately run out there too. So I suspected that six weeks in and six weeks out could only end in permanently 'in', and inevitably it would be without warning—and a bed one had been counting on would suddenly and permanently be filled. I had already had enough headaches myself, running a summer holiday relief system on a much more limited scale for a much more limited time. It had all the complications of a hotel booking system but with the added worry that one would collect several unexpected and permanent guests on the way—beds would not be free in time—so that much heartburning recriminations and suffering would ensue.

The layers of habitual and traditional thought had not then been peeled away! This was a traditional practice—everybody did it—it was a needed public service. As an admitting doctor, it was always pleasant to clerk in a 'custodial care' patient—one subconsciously relaxed one's standards—one knew this was a patient going home again in two weeks' time—the main thing was to make sure that he went home at least as well as he had come in. His stay was to be made as comfortable as possible but there was no need to fall over backward to remobilise him or try to encourage independence, if it was not there spontaneously. In a sense, it was a 'left luggage' service, with the parcel having to be delivered back in the same state as it had been deposited.

Sometimes, when revisiting such families the following year, it amazed me that a good time never seemed to have been had by all. On occasion, I was even more astonished to be visiting households at crisis point not very long after a 'Good' holiday had been supposedly had by the family. Daughters would say, "Dad was very difficult when he got back from hospital and it took him a long time to settle down again. I sometimes wonder if it was worth it, but" (desperately), "hubby and the children do need to get away for a holiday and I must study them occasionally".

The custodial system of holiday admission for just over two weeks at a time was used at Edgware until the year there were 300 requests for holiday relief. When this was appreciated and the requests analysed and it was found in fact that only 32 of these people actually needed to be in hospital for medical and nursing support, then some agonising reappraisal went on. It was felt that when a thing had got so out of hand and become hopelessly impractical, then basic thinking needed revision.

One of the fantastic elements in the situation was found to be that requests were being received from doctors and relatives in November to book a place for their patient in a hospital bed the following August.

CONUNDRUM

Question	When is a hospital not a hospital?
Answer	When it is being used as a hotel.

SUBSIDIARY

Question	Why do you say it is being used as a hotel?
Answer	Only a necromancer, or a very specially gifted doctor indeed, can say in November the year previously that a patient is going to need to be in hospital between specified dates the following August.

Question Is this always the case?

Answer No. It is possible that the patient may have considerable disability or disease at the time of the referral in November, in which case he needs to be in hospital in November, not waiting for ten months before he goes in.

Question Are you then saying that relatives do not deserve holidays?

Answer No. I consider that everyone needs a holiday, and longer ones than are usually taken, and I particularly consider that older people need a change from their long-suffering relatives—for what can be more painful than living with someone who is long-suffering for fifty weeks of the year.

But levity aside, this is probably the most emotive question in the book of personal relationships—chiefly because the community social resources are far behind the actual needs.

The higher average standards of living mean that many more people are going away on holidays—going further and for longer periods. This is a social custom and right of today. It was not the custom or right of the majority of the population a few decades ago: a day at Blackpool or Southend was often the total extent of holiday away for the average working man or woman. This means, therefore, that the people who are causing their families concern—the 70 and 80-year-olds—are not viewing holidays in quite the same light and are *ipso facto* less concerned whether they or the family do go away.

For much the same reasons, they themselves are not as keen on travelling long distances for long periods. Understandably too, many older people find no great interest in noisy seaside resorts or in travelling to places where there is very hot sun; the journeys themselves are tedious and exhausting and strange tongues, sights, customs and food are harder to assimilate for short periods. What is more acceptable is either to go to a quieter place nearer home or preferably to remain at home, receiving, from an alternative source, support normally given by the absent family.

It is the alternative quiet residential accommodation or the alternative support that is often so sadly in short supply. For too long, hospitals have been filling the social gap and in the process, perhaps, demoralising quite a number of elderly people. What holiday can it have been for them to spend two weeks in hospital—would you like to do this voluntarily yourself? Some abnegatory souls can be heard to murmur, "Yes, if it would enable my devoted daughter/son to go away and enjoy their holiday in peace."

But is this the answer? Is it not yet again forcing our elderly kith and kin to acquiesce in distress to what is available rather than making a fuss and ensuring that something more appropriate is made available, and soon?

Let me relate 84-year-old *MRS. MILLINER'S* triumph in this direction. But first let us review the map on page 12 (***Figure*** 3). Roxbourne Hospital (ex-isolation hospital) has been one of the Geriatric Unit hospitals for some fifteen years or more, but still it is looked on by the local population and, even more regrettably (such is the slowness of receptive communication in medical circles), by many of the general practitioners in the area as, alternatively, an Old People's Home or else a private nursing home.

It is usually referred to as "Roxborough Nursing Home". It is not surprising, therefore, that Mrs. Milliner's story, as far as we are concerned, opens with a certificate from her family doctor certifying Mrs. Milliner's need for custodial care from September 6th to the 20th next, addressed to the matron of 'Roxborough Nursing Home'.

This information was supplemented by subsequent conversation between the matron and Mrs. Milliner's daughter, the substance of which the matron transmitted to the main Geriatric Administrative Office at Edgware where all the requests are dealt with. The supplementary information stated that Mrs. Milliner had had a stroke the previous November, leaving her with a right hemiplegia. She was bedridden, but not incontinent and could be got into a chair with help. She had not had any kind of rehabilitation. The daughter was single and out at work all day, and had tried to get someone to look after her mother so that she could take a holiday, but had had no success.

Even on this information, the physician who does the day-today administrative work commented that a much more constructive approach could have been made to a patient who remained continent despite eight months in bed and who had a right hemiplegia. This same physician made the home visit about a week later and made a footnote on the report of the visit that the daughter stated that when she went to see the family doctor to ask him to arrange admission for the patient, he had seemed very cross about the whole business! One wonders why. It seemed a very reasonable request—but perhaps he was annoyed that it had not been made sooner!

The hospital doctor learned that the patient not only had a right hemiplegia but her right leg had been crippled since she had been knocked over by a bicycle when she was a child. She had a fixed right knee and had worn a built-up shoe at one time but in later years had discarded it. In consequence, her left knee and hip were almost permanently flexed to accommodate for the shortening of the right leg. A nice technical problem this.

Socially, she was a widow and the daughter was the breadwinner; the daughter was away from home from 7.15 am to 5.30 pm and two good neighbours took it in turns to come in and give a midday meal and toilet aid. From 5.30 pm on and at the weekends the daughter managed single-handed. She had a particularly exacting job and had to work in a dark room all day. She was approaching retirement age herself. One scarcely needs to labour the point that Miss Milliner led a pretty circumscribed life and the holiday was much needed. The relationship between mother and daughter, however, was excellent and they were both delighted at my colleague's suggestion that Mrs. Milliner needed to come into hospital, not for custodial care but in her own right, to see whether she could regain independence. The holiday was of secondary importance, for in all probability it might take longer than the holiday to get Mrs. Milliner back on her feet; if this proved to be so, the daughter would be able to go away quite happily.

In the event, it took nearly four months to get her independent enough to go to Springbok House, our convalescent annexe or half-way house. By then, she had been equipped with a hearing aid (miraculous in itself, for nowadays it takes many weeks to have an appointment with the ENT Department—it then takes about five months to obtain the actual aid from the Hearing Aid Centre) and also a below-knee iron for her weak right leg, with a special supporting mechanism for the old injured knee. She used a walking frame to support herself and give her more confidence when walking along open spaces, such as the long hospital ward or corridor. She remained at Springbok for two weeks—long enough to regain her 'sea legs'—and home she went. Soon after her return home she had bronchitis and pleurisy but this only kept her in bed for a day or two. Three weeks later she appeared in the follow-up clinic, bright as a button and wearing such a superb millinery concoction that old hospital friends were summoned to see her, and it, and much gaiety was added to a somewhat grim February day.

That year there was no request for admission to hospital. Mrs. Milliner went on holiday herself to one of the Welfare Authority's residential Homes which was out in the country. Next year she had an attack of shingles and more bronchitis (it was an old house and very difficult to keep warm in the winter) but she did not have to go to bed—she stayed up and about, using her walking frame and helping with the household chores. Again during that year there was a holiday for Mrs. Milliner as well as the daughter.

Then came this year. For some reason, perhaps her own impending retirement at the end of the year, Miss Milliner did not request holiday accommodation soon enough for her mother, and a query from the Welfare Department as to whether she wanted help (which took the form of a telephone message to her at her place of work) was not delivered.

The first we knew of this was a call from the family doctor asking us to take the patient in for a period of custodial care (as remarked before, receptive communication is a slow process).

Mrs. Milliner and Miss Milliner were both extremely perturbed on learning that there was no prospect of accommodation at one of the local Welfare Homes, and Mrs. Milliner was so upset on her daughter's behalf that our medical social worker took emergency action and found a vacancy in a Red Cross Holiday Home. The next thing we knew was a telephone call from Miss Milliner to say that her mother had collapsed in the garden, with severe abdominal pain, and had been rushed into her nearest hospital—which, despite Mrs. Milliner's pleas, was not ours. Knowing Mrs. Milliner's recent stress and her general tendency, our doctors muttered "constipation" amongst themselves and did not worry unduly, but Mrs. Milliner developed bronchopneumonia as well and died shortly after. Even so, I think one could postulate that she had almost died 'with her boots on'.

Equally, I think it would be fair to postulate that if she had been admitted as requested three years previously for a two-week period of custodial care and left in bed all the time and the next year admitted again for two weeks' care, long before another year had passed or even before then, she would have become a long-stay patient. For how long could her daughter have supported this situation? I think, in fact, with the further information gleaned since the event, the daughter was nearer cracking point than we had imagined when we were first invited to help. It transpired that there had been many difficulties at work and one of the neighbours we had thought "so good" was actually a source of great difficulty because she was so indispensable to the fabric of the support of the household that she tended to take advantage of the situation, and both mother and daughter were miserably under her domination. This is not an extreme example; this is an all too common example of the sort of situation one finds when visiting following a request for custodial care. Sometimes the referring doctor adds a little rider to the request, such as, "What a good family this is and how well they have coped with this very difficult problem for so long." One longs to cry, "You're too right, cobber", but this would be too hurtful to too many genuinely concerned practitioners who, like oneself a few years ago, had not had the layers of habitual thought peeled away.

> "'Tis just like a summer bird-cage in a garden;
> the birds that are without despair to get in,
> and the birds that are within despair and are in
> a consumption for fear they shall never get out."
>
> *John Webster*

References

1. Binks, F. Allen. (1964). *Lancet,* **ii,** 1233-36.
2. *'Stroke/Counterstroke'.* Film comparing modern methods of team work with Douglas Ritchie's lonely struggle to rehabilitate. Produced by Smith, Kline & French (Drugs), at Edgware General Hospital, 1967.

Chapter Five

FUNCTION

"The temporary passive acceptance which is all that is needed from the patient for the efficacy of intravenous therapy or radiotherapy, for example, is often not differentiated from the continuous participation with intent, purpose and motive which is essential if physiotherapy and occupational therapy are to be effective".[1]

We have already considered the limitations of physiotherapy in connection with the redoubtable Mrs. Crier (*page* 23) who had no motivation towards independence so resisted all attempts, even the recommended 'force' in learning to walk again. But what are the bounds of physical therapy and how should it be used? Should short courses of exercise therapy be given, stopped and then started again three months later, as is so often recommended? Or should there be long-term, purposeful activity on the part of the therapist, to match as closely as possible the need of the patient at the time?

Couched in this way, the question answers itself and one wonders a little why there should be such widely divergent views. The paramount consideration lies in what people mean by physiotherapy. In many patients' minds 'physiotherapist' is just a superior name for masseuse and a masseuse is a wonderful lady who first warms the painful part and will then tenderly massage it, meanwhile listening to the patient's troubles and saying reassuring things. There is undoubtedly a tremendous aching void here that only the Japanese seem to have filled adequately with their Geisha tea gardens. It would be interesting to do a spot check on some of the central London physiotherapy departments and note just how many tense, high-powered executives who have bad backs—lumbago, sciatica, slipped discs and so on—find their way unwittingly to the Physical Medicine Departments and so to a course of physiotherapy. This tremendous primitive urge to have one's stresses smoothed away is only too understandable.

And is this why physiotherapists are no longer called masseuses? I am told by my physiotherapy colleagues that nowadays it is rare to be told to give a patient massage, although in the teaching of students it still has a place in the syllabus.

Lackaday! Physiotherapy has gone the way of all the professional medical disciplines: it has become as scientific as the rest, heat, light and sound now being the order of the day, with quantities of brisk exercises too. These days, the only time there seems to be any laying on of hands is in the performance of intricate manipulative techniques. Final insult— the most modern physiotherapists clap ice on the painful parts—so now we have to contend with a quadruple, heat, light, sound and cold. But perhaps in many ways this is more compatible with our climate, for it is a worrying sight to see patients queueing up at a freezing bus stop for twenty to thirty minutes when one knows they have only recently come away from the Out-Patient Department where they have been lying under a heat lamp for a quarter of an hour or so to ease their aches and pains. The other extreme is the arthritic who may travel miles on a scorching hot summer's day in order to immerse her hands in a wax bath. A book of Graham Greene's left a query in my mind.[2] It was about a leprosarium in French Equatorial Africa where everything and everybody was wilting in the humid heat and a devoted doctor was railing against the powers that be who had not despatched adequate equipment to help him treat his disabled lepers. One of the bits of equipment he wanted was a wax bath!

I think it is true that arthritics do gain by this treatment, particularly very disabled and housebound rheumatoid arthritics, and I am very sure they benefit; they have told me when I have seen them at home how much they have missed the outing to hospital twice or thrice weekly. When pressed for explanation of benefit, they would usually pinpoint it fairly spontaneously, commenting that it is the only chance they have of seeing the outside world.

The epitome of this form of palliative therapy is an elderly couple I met whilst visiting the wife's mother at home. They are both osteo-arthritics and they attend a famous clinic in London. They were highly indignant when that clinic closed and they were temporarily deviated to their local hospital a quarter of a mile away. Their outing to town together once a week was a regular feature of their lives. The hospital transport car took them and as it was the same car each time, I have no doubt that they had reached some companionable agreement about stopping en route for shopping. Their resentment was such, life must have been uncomfortable in many places until the clinic opened again in new quarters and took them on the list once more.

But this is the same old story. A genuine social need is being distorted and hidden by the use of therapy and treatment. The very conditions we have imposed invite people to create or perpetuate physical complaints so that they can continue to receive the social support that they need and have finally obtained (inappropriately) by attendance at some hospital Out-Patient Department. This is all too frequently the Physical Medicine Department (PMD), for, like the Geriatric Department, the PMD is used by colleagues when they can think of nothing more to do with difficult and unrewarding patients who ungratefully refuse to respond to other therapy. To wit, the difficult Mrs. Crier (*page* 23) who had been wished on to the PMD as an out-patient by the medical firm who would have nothing more to do with her. Fortunately for themselves, however, very few PMD's have beds allocated to them, so that fairly incisive action is possible without fear of having to accept ultimate long-term responsibility.

Having said all this, if there are any physiotherapists amongst my readers, they will be wondering why we consider it important to have any on our re-ablement team. Here again, one needs a qualitative analysis. Just as we need a nurse or a doctor or a social worker, it cannot be *any* of these, but only particular ones, who are of like minds and compatible temperaments. An authoritarian, insensitive person, disinterested in the reasons and causes for disability and preoccupied with the technicalities of 'treatment' would be as useless to us as a talking parrot, and probably more harmful.

There is a great need, amongst the patients, for people who

thoroughly understand their locomotor problems, who can work out from first principles of anatomy, coupled with their knowledge and experience of disease, where the troubles lie and how they can best be overcome. This requires not only a sound basic training and an informed objective critical faculty but a logical, orderly mind to break down physical disabilities into their component parts, and strengthen and reinforce what remains and re-train to a different pattern where necessary.

A small example of this came to my notice not long since. The husband of a niece of a patient of ours came to one of our Relatives' Conferences. He was an extremely fit, proud man who had suffered a stroke not long after his aunt-in-law. He had regained power rapidly, but had needed to go on wearing a leg-iron, which he demonstrated to us. We were puzzled why this was necessary when he had such excellent dorsiflexion of his foot, but undoubtedly he did catch his toe when he walked. Several physiotherapists had had dealings with him and many were the reasons that had been suggested, but it was our team physiotherapist who applied first principles and studied his walking pattern. It was noted that he had, for some reason during his re-training, developed a habit of never fully straightening his opposite knee when that leg was taking weight in walking, so that the affected leg never had the full length to 'swing through'. When he corrected this tendency to bend the good knee, he had no further trouble.

Perhaps some more illustrations of how physiotherapists fit into the team would be of greater value than any further general observations.

There was *MRS. GOER* who was 78 when our paths first crossed. She was referred from the surgeons in the laconic terms, "Fractured shaft of femur; varicose ulcer; daughter cannot manage her at home; I don't think she will walk again; please advise re disposal".

A technical problem once more. And in due course Mrs. Goer was transferred to one of the sadly-named chronic surgical beds. Let us fill in the background to Mrs. Goer a little. She had been widowed when young, brought up her daughter single handed and had held a responsible job. She lived with her daughter and son-in-law (the latter retired) and was a loved and respected member of the household. Prior to admission (which was five months before her transfer) she had been able to walk on the flat, using two tripod walking sticks; these had been necessary because she had severe osteo-arthritis of her hips. She had spent two and a half years confined to the first floor of her daughter's house because this was where the lavatory and bathroom were and she insisted on being independent. She had fallen on the landing on her way back from the bathroom one day and had fractured the upper third of her femoral shaft.

When she arrived on our ward her disabilities were great, from a structural point of view—2 inches shortening, very little movement in her hips, a big varicose ulcer on the affected side; an apprehensive and somewhat demoralised woman who saw no future for herself apart from a dependent wheel-chair existence.

Apart from the doctor and nurse, the next member of the team to get to know Mrs. Goer was the physiotherapist—a single-handed part timer. She cheerfully suggested that they should try walking together. Mrs. Goer was terribly apprehensive, but co-operative, although she expressed surprise as she was not used to doing such things on the ward. She had always had to undergo an exhausting trip to the gymnasium before and queued up, waiting her turn. She had always been supported by two physiotherapists and doubted whether one would be adequate to prevent her falling.

She did not fall, and with the physiotherapist's stalwart encouragement, she was soon walking independently once more, with a walking frame for support, after which they worked out together the height of bed and chair she needed and how and where—either in bed or on the chair—dressing was best accomplished. During this period the physiotherapist learnt more about Mrs. Goer's background and heard about the family and saw the daughter when she was visiting. She was then able to report that as far as the family were concerned, they were only too ready to have Mrs. Goer back and as soon as possible, though it would be more practical if she were able to do as much for herself as she had been doing before the accident.

This news gave fresh impetus to the effort and thought being given by the physiotherapist to the problem of doing stairs. It was found that Mrs. Goer had not enough hip flexion to manage stairs in the ordinary way, but by tipping her pelvis she could manage a step of 4 inches. Our occupational therapy colleagues then came into the picture and made a half-step of 4 inches and as the stair rise at home was 8 inches, by an intricate and rather stately side-square step, it was found to be possible for Mrs. Goer to climb the stairs at home once more, unaided. Only the ulceration of her leg was left to hinder her discharge from hospital. By using the weekly dressing, with medicated bandage technique, its enormous proportions were reduced considerably, but we wanted it completely healed before she left us.

She went home four months after transfer to us—nine months after admission to hospital. Apart from her healed ulcer, Mrs. Goer's disabilities had not altered in any way, but her function had increased beyond measure. There was no magic in this; the only real key had been entirely in the attitude and approach. Someone had taken the trouble to find out the family's true attitude. From there it was purely a matter of encouragement (and Barkis was more than willing!) and mechanics.

This episode had sequel after sequel. Mrs. Goer always attributed her success to the marvellous staff, particularly the physiotherapist concerned, and at a time when unpleasant letters were appearing in the press about the way old folk were treated, she decided this was not good enough and wrote a letter to the local paper. There was no doubt that beauty lay in the eye of the beholder, for she heaped all praise possible on the wonderful treatment she had had from the Occupational Therapy Department. We were puzzled, as she knew us all well; the occupational therapists were highly embarrassed, for, apart from the actual making of the half-step, they had, for once, not been involved in this particular problem. The explanation was soon forthcoming from Mrs. Goer herself when I asked her obliquely about it on one of her periodic visits. As she had remained on the ward doing only ordinary things after being transferred to us and had never again gone to the gymnasium or done many formal exercises or had any specific treatment apart from dressings for her leg, she had decided that the physiotherapists must have abandoned her to the occupational therapists, and though her uniform was unlike the others, our physiotherapist must really have been an OT in disguise.

Her life at home was one of expansion, not contraction, and she frequently said how she blessed the day she broke her leg. For one thing, she found that the terrible joint pains she had had previously had all disappeared—did we think it was due to the electric bed (ripple alternating air cell mattress to prevent pressure sores) she was on when she first came into hospital?!

We had visualised her climbing up and down stairs once a day but with the aid of her half-step she was going up and down when the spirit (and nature) moved her. She had gone out for a picnic for the first time in three years and her joy in the smell of grass was a morale-raiser in itself. Then, because she had heard someone saying at a Relatives' Conference how we wished that walking frames could be made as common a sight in the street as tripod walking sticks (and then people would not be embarrassed to use them out-of-doors), she started taking short strolls up and down her road with her walking frame, and was consequently able to re-discover the pleasure of being able to call on her friends. Such a change, she remarked, to be able to visit them instead of having to wait for them to come and see her.

At another Relatives' Conference, the subject came up of allowing people to live dangerously and independently, and Mrs. Goer's daughter suddenly held forth. She and her husband were anxious to visit their children—one in Africa and one in America. How could they possibly do so unless they knew that Mrs. Goer was being adequately cared for? There was a tremendous chorus of support when Mrs. Goer said she was perfectly capable of looking after herself, and we agreed. The daughter buttonholed us again after the meeting to make sure we really meant this. In due course, they went off on their holiday, leaving a cousin of similar age to Mrs. Goer in the house with her. We did not learn until long after the holiday was over that Mrs. Goer had cunningly said that the hospital had insisted that she was to spend at least one week on her own; the last week she had indeed had on her own and enjoyed every minute of it. A further interesting technical point is that despite the apparent and permanent limitation in

Mrs. Goer's hip movement, in the fullness of time she was not only going up and downstairs frequently; she was able also to dispense with the raised lavatory seat she had needed when she first went home. Another instance, perhaps, of mobility breeding greater mobility.

One can see, as she often says, "Life is much sweeter than before the fracture".

The case is a very specialised one but it is a good demonstration of team-work: it demonstrates not skilled techniques or magical formulae but how, if there is determination on the part of the patient and a willingness to slog on endlessly on the part of the professionals, plus goodwill and support from the family, then even the seemingly impossible can be achieved.

The reverse side of the coin was *MRS. WILHOLM,* akin to Mrs. Goer because she too was endowed with a leonine courage and a determination which called forth similar qualities from all who came into contact with her. 'Not possible' and 'Can't' were not part of her vocabulary and never had been. She was 73 when we met her and to relate even a fragment of the transactions that ensued requires a chapter of its own.

"And wilt thou leave me thus? Say nay,
say nay, for shame!"

Sir Thomas Wyatt

References

1. Binks, F. Allen. (1968). *Brit. Med. J.,* **i**, 269-74.
2. Greene, Graham. (1961). "*A Burnt-Out Case*". *London. W. Heinemann Ltd. Price* 16*s*. 0*d*.

Chapter Six

FUNCTION *(continued)*

> *"Diseases desperate grown, by desperate appliances are relieved, or not at all."*
> *William Shakespeare, Hamlet, IV. iii.* 9

Mrs. Wilholm had a very interested and good family doctor who rang us after the Christmas recess to request "an out-patient appointment for assessment and advice". Mrs. Wilholm, he reported, had been discharged from an 'acute' medical ward a week before Christmas. She had been there nineteen weeks for treatment of congestive heart failure. She was a 'burnt-out' rheumatoid arthritic and her heart failure had been put right by bed rest, but she was now unable to stand alone. She was at her daughter's flat and accommodation was inadequate. She had her own flat, but her doctor felt that she was past caring for herself.

We found her old hospital notes before going to see her, as we felt that with this history a trip to a hospital's Out-Patient Department in the middle of winter could only be detrimental. The old notes reported the gruesome details of her breathlessness nine weeks before admission, and her ultimate capitulation in agreeing to come into hospital after several frightening attacks of breathlessness at night. It was small wonder that she was frightened because both her parents and four of her brothers and sisters had died with heart trouble. It is curious too, looking back on things, that when one considers the subsequent physical efforts she made during her time with us, she never had any further trouble with her heart and never required any further treatment for it. She had been known to have rheumatoid arthritis for some thirty years and there was an entry in the notes suggesting that it would be a good idea for her to have a session in the Functional Assessment Unit when she was fit enough and before discharge home, and that diversional occupational therapy should be started. There was no record that this was done, nor was there any record in the medical notes of her social background or her physical function. She was, in traditional terms, a 'heart case'; once she had been treated for the condition for which she was admitted to hospital, she was discharged home.

Knowing Mrs. Wilholm's particular personality, I have no doubt that she put no obstacles in the way. That she had not been out of bed for eighteen weeks, or dressed or walked, would have been of small moment to her; she would expect to be able to do this once she got safely home to her own surroundings and could order things as she pleased. There was, too, that judgment-warping festival about to occur—Christmas.

It is a never failing source of amazement to me (and I shall soon be celebrating my 21st hospital Christmas) how Christmas, and to a lesser extent other religious and Bank Holidays, affects people both inside and outside hospital.

Inside hospital there is a united feeling from patients and staff—shut down; empty the wards; get home as fast as possible. No one wants to come in from the waiting lists: an unofficial moratorium is declared. The only wards that are really and genuinely upset if there is no work are the maternity, particularly the labour wards, and the children's wards. On the other hand, the geriatric wards are subjected to the most paradoxical pressures from within and without. Patients whom one knows are not well enough to go home, and who have totally unwelcoming domestic circumstances, press desperately to be discharged. From the outside world, there is a sudden upsurge of pleas for help, from all sorts of unexpected sources, for the destitute and deserving. This is hardly surprising when one considers the way we conduct our national Christmas holiday. For almost a week, all the community services close down and only a sprinkling of emergency staff are on duty anywhere. Coupled with this is the flurry of pre-Christmas activity on the part of voluntary organisations and people of goodwill visiting the old, the needy and the neglected. There is the giving out of coal vouchers, groceries, gift parcels and Christmas 'cheer'. In the process it is inevitable that small pockets of unsuspected squalor and misery are brought to light, and naturally those making such discovery are unable to rest and enjoy their own Christmas, unless they can be assured that something has been done to alleviate the horror they have found. The 'something' usually takes the form of admission to hospital.

All in all, one can see why it was that Mrs. Wilholm went home the week before Christmas, treated for the condition which brought her into hospital but without her capabilities for independent living having been fully re-tried and despite her daughter's protestations and warnings that she was not yet ready.

To describe the personality of Mrs. Wilholm would require the talents of a Somerset Maugham. I can only relate the few facts that we came to know of her past and then relate them to her present with us.

She had been widowed in the 1914-18 War and had brought up her family of three daughters single handed. In due course, they had married and left home, and seventeen years previously Mrs. Wilholm had been allocated one of the Council's old people's flatlets. This was in a small close, tucked away behind the main roads and quite a walk from the shops. The basic design of the flat was reasonable enough—an L-shaped bed-sitting room, the short arm of which could be curtained off as a sleeping area—the kitchen opened off the living end and there was a small lobby entrance with a w.c. leading off it. The snags were—an open fire, a bath under a wooden cover in the kitchen and a high step and lintel to the front door which opened on to a covered way, about 4 feet wide, from which there were two steep steps down into a little garden. Mrs. Wilholm loved her garden, and having been disabled for a long time, she had already reconstructed this so that she, and it, could meet at a workable level. She had tubs and window boxes and troughs raised on trestles, and all around and scattered between were handy boxes used as platforms and seats for resting whilst working and walking, for she had been using two elbow crutches for some years.

The arthritis we knew was of thirty years' duration, but some ten years prior to our advent on the scene she had been involved in a motor accident. The car in which she was travelling had to brake suddenly and she had been thrown forward, striking her chin on the seat in front, her head being jerked backwards. Following this incident she had begun to lose the power in her legs, becoming unsteady when walking and unable to dig her garden. This last caused her to seek medical advice, and she was investigated with great thoroughness at one of the big hospitals for nervous diseases in London. There, after much deliberation, it was decided that she had evidence of proximal wasting and weakness in her lower limbs, suggesting a proximal form of myopathy, for which no definite cause could be found. There was no evidence of carcinoma or endocrine disease. She had cervical spondylosis and the car-jolting incident had precipitated more trouble. They recommended that she should have physiotherapy at her local hospital, and that was that.

Mrs. Wilholm had a little physiotherapy, collected her crutches and decided that the best thing was to live as normally as she could: she did not bother much further with the medical fraternity! Her daughter saw to her more difficult cleaning chores and got any shopping that was not delivered, and Mrs. Wilholm's neighbours, with whom she was on very good terms, supplemented the rest.

Retrospectively, out of our own knowledge of the area, it is conceivable to postulate some of the reasons that may have upset the even tenor of Mrs. Wilholm's life and have led to her nineteen-week hospital stay. One of the features of that year had been the abominable summer and spring, following on a miserable winter and a poor summer the year before. We had noted a rising incidence of morbidity during that autumn, at an unexpected period. We attributed it to the fact that many of our frailer and more handicapped patients had hardly been out of doors for a twelve month or more, and the approach of winter and the known ensiegement it brought, without having the benefit of re-charging their life batteries in the warm fresh air, had produced a tremendous failure of morale. It is very important for anyone doing this sort of work to pay particular attention to the weather—particularly the onset of the really cold and frosty times—each year; for several weeks and months later, one is seeing people at home who have taken to their beds at a particular time for no explicable physical reason. Often with careful but nonchalant questioning one can establish that a virtual hibernation has occurred, and if this proves to be so, a much happier prognosis can be given.

This, then, could have been an influential factor in Mrs. Wilholm's deterioration, for she had loved being out in her garden. Another was probably related to her neighbours. There were six flats on the ground floor of her block and we had been called to see one of her neighbours previously. This was *MRS. BETHNAL*—a 90-year-old in a very sordid, neglected, miserable state, suffering from gross myxoedema and mortal fear. She was a tough old cockney, alone in the world with her cat, Jack, and in fear because *her* next-door-neighbour had been found lying cold and dead the day previously and had obviously been so for some time without anybody knowing. Would this be her fate too? Two other neighbours had also died unexpectedly and she suddenly felt very lonely and frightened. In fact, she came into hospital (her doctor and his family took over her cat, for she refused to budge until Jack was cared for), responded well to treatment of her myxoedema and to tender loving care, and after a spell at Springbok House, insisted that she was now going home. This meant heroic efforts from social agencies, both voluntary and statutory, as winter was just beginning, but all went well and she has flourished exceedingly. In fact, her life is fuller than before, though unhappily Jack was lost and a substitute had to be found (all part and parcel of the process of re-ablement!). However, no doubt gloom at the deaths and Mrs. Bethnal's sudden departure to the Geriatric Ward had all taken their toll of Mrs. Wilholm and had in all probability played a part in her original breakdown and hospital admission.

To return to Mrs. Wilholm's saga, home she went and the first night, getting out to the w.c. she slipped and fell, and her daughter found her lying on the floor next day, frozen and exhausted. The family doctor felt reluctant to ask for further help from the hospital when she had just come home after nineteen weeks' stay, and in all probability Mrs. Wilholm would have refused to return. So the daughter took her back to her own two-bedroomed flat. She and her husband turned out of their bed and room and slept on a put-u-up settee in their only living room, but as they had two adult sons still living at home, space was very cramped. There was, however, no shortage of goodwill.

Mrs. Wilholm herself at that time was very depressed by her

helplessness and frustrated by her dependence on her daughter. Despite her hand deformities, she was doing some beautiful embroidery. In bed, she was able to move herself about quite well by her own method of dragging herself along on her elbows. Standing, however, was not possible as she was quite unable to fix her trunk on her legs, so to speak, long enough to walk with her crutches. We felt that even with *her* spirit, walking would not be possible but she could, perhaps, achieve wheel-chair independence. Knowing, from our previous visit to Mrs. Bethnal the type of flat in which she lived, we thought it unlikely that she would be able to manage there again, but this thought Mrs. Wilholm brushed aside. She wanted to get into hospital and get to work on walking practice.

And this is where the battle began, primarily for the physiotherapist and nurses, who were first in the line of fire, but ultimately for a greater section of the hospital and outside community services than we have ever experienced before or since. There was a very simple reason for this : Mrs. Wilholm wished to go home to her own flat and take up living there, where she had left off—on her own. *Full stop*. She was a resourceful woman herself who had always supplemented her pension, even when disabled, by making all sorts of soft goods, toys, ornaments, artificial flowers and anything in vogue or requested, and she obviously felt that as we were trained professionals, we should be able to do just as well, if not better.

At first things seemed to be going well and she managed to walk hanging on to the parallel bars. We had hopes of a walking aid, but then suddenly complete flaccid paralysis occurred and, worse still from her point of view, she lost bladder control. In a sense, this was very useful, as it was then reasonable to use an indwelling catheter, and at least one of her potential hazards was eliminated : her urine would drain into a disposable plastic bag and she would not have to get out at night to spend a penny. This fresh incident confirmed our neurologist's opinion that her condition was probably due to a myelopathy of vascular origin. Her legs became oedematous and completely paralysed and a great weight and nuisance for a time; so much so, that, seeing a legless lady of 87 getting herself from bed to wheel-chair fairly easily,

Mrs. Wilholm suggested very seriously that we should summon the surgeons and ask them to amputate her legs.

At this stage we were definitely feeling that all hope of home would have to be abandoned and Mrs. Wilholm would have to settle for wheel-chair independence and allow an application to be made for her admission to a designated residential Home, i.e. where simple nursing help is provided. This was put to her by the medical social worker, and after sleeping on it, she asked if she might first spend a day at home, reviewing the situation. As she pointed out, by this time she had hardly been in her home for six months.

This seemed an excellent idea, and I for one thought it would settle the matter; she would find how impossible it was for her to manage and we could take it from there. Arrangements were made—her daughter would have the place warm and everything ready—the ambulance would deliver Mrs. Wilholm mid-morning—she and daughter could have lunch together—the hospital team would arrive mid-afternoon to see the flat, find out what had happened and have an on site discussion.

And so it came to pass; we even took along our cine camera to record things. We still have the record. Far from deciding to give up, Mrs. Wilholm was even more determined to go home. When she had demonstrated her abilities, by making tea for us all and washing-up, despite the disparate heights of wheel-chair, sink and working surfaces, we had to agree too, that somehow it should be possible. One can only admit to a feeling of intense selfish gloom, for stretching before one was a vista of unremitting hard endeavour before things could be so manipulated as to make anything nearly adequate for Mrs. Wilholm's return, and the department generally had so many things on its communal plate and so many things screaming to be done. There was, however, no help for it—the physiotherapist was quietly confident that somewhere, somehow, it should be possible to find a hoist Mrs. Wilholm could use, and was duly measuring the sleeping area and doorways. At the same time the occupational therapist was measuring up heights in the kitchen and the camera was whirring. Mrs. Wilholm looked happily confident too of our capabilities although her daughter appeared terror-struck at the enormity of the whole thing.

Time passed, Mrs. Wilholm pressed, but when it was firmly laid down that certain criteria had to be fulfilled before she could go home, she saw the point. The first and most important objective was that she must be able to transfer from bed to chair or commode and *vice versa*, entirely unaided, either under her own steam or with self-operated mechanical help. However, after much trial and despite all Mrs. Wilholm's physical exertions, the problem of raising her heavy flaccid legs remained unsolved and a hoist was decided upon. The problem of her passing urine was more or less settled, for, although catheterisation had been difficult and there had been a lot of blood in her urine for a time, this had settled and the catheter was working. The problem of bowel action had not been solved; this was really a problem as she had always tended towards constipation and since her paralysis this had become severe; she had on occasion taken sixteen laxative tablets without result!

Bowel habit had to be predictably regulated as she would be dependent upon the district nurse to empty her commode, for, owing to the structure of the flat, she could not manoeuvre her wheel-chair into the lavatory, nor could any structural alteration be made to enable her to do so.

So there was a very basic problem—and how often bowels are so. The nurses worked hard on this one and eventually it was found that by a judicious use of laxative tablets the night before and the use of a suppository, her bowels would act in twenty minutes, giving her time to hoist herself on to a commode or bedpan.

Meanwhile, the physiotherapist had been immersed in literature and enquiries and discussions, had worked out the best type of hoist and immediately ran into the usual hitches—money, and the fact that Mrs. Wilholm lived in a council flat. Therefore any structural alterations or fixtures were virtually ruled out. The hoist had to be self-operating and so designed that it would lift her high enough to ensure that her flaccid, heavy legs and dangling feet cleared the edge of the bed. Following some rather hilarious demonstrations from various hoist firms, it was eventually decided that the best combination was a simple block and tackle with a traverse bar, fixed to a wonderful free-standing superstructure that the hospital engineers had rigged with gas piping and fixed to a hospital bedstead.

Having found this method, the problem of slings then arose, as Mrs. Wilholm was anaesthetic below her waist and it was important that the slings should have no selvedged edge to damage her skin. All the known slings had this edge, but eventually fire hose was thought of and the husband of one of our *REABLISTS** was dispatched to the local Fire Station for some old fire hose. Someone else knew someone with a commercial type sewing machine and the slings were made. At the same time thought had to be given to many other problems, such as disposal of space-occupying furniture, telephone installation, gas cooker and working surface heights, lowering of gas water heater and sink and trying to have the useless bath removed from the kitchen, organising voluntary visitors for shopping, etc.

During all these multitudinous trials and arrangements, which were inevitably done via telephones, writing and interviews, not involving the patient, there was, from her point of view, a hiatus. During this hiatus she withdrew into herself, turned her face literally to the wall and looked broken and dejected like a rag doll out of which the stuffing had run. It took a little time for us to realise the cause, but she soon perked up when she knew we had not simply abandoned her without letting her know, but had the work well in hand. Contrary to the old adage, it seems necessary to go about one's work more noisily than training recommends!

By then we felt we had more or less completed our side and the time had come to foregather with daughter, the welfare officers concerned with the handicapped, and the district nurse. For, we thought, all that was now needed was for the Welfare Department to duplicate the hoist at home and arrange certain adaptations to the kitchen, have a telephone installed and, if possible, a ramp. Ramps took a long time and we had warned Mrs. Wilholm that she would be a prisoner in her flat for a lengthy period. She said she would be happy as long as she could open her front door and smell the fresh air and look at her garden.

Now some of the greatest frustrations occurred, both for us and for Mrs. Wilholm. Firstly, there was a rule in her borough

*Reablists see page 148

that no alterations could be made or apparatus or help provided until a person was registered as physically handicapped. Secondly, such registration had to be made in the person's own home and not in hospital. Deadlock. A nice 'Alice through the Looking Glass' touch this seemed. To go home, Mrs. Wilholm had to have alterations and equipment; these could not even be put to a Committee until she was registered, and even then time had to elapse—permission had to be granted, tenders obtained and work carried out. Worse still, the welfare personnel concerned were all too busy to come to the hospital and meet the patient and talk about it. We had two failures before we eventually persuaded them to come to the FAC, the daughter having taken time off work each time. The moment they met Mrs. Wilholm and saw her demonstrate her capabilities of transferring from bed to chair, get herself about in her chair and so on, difficulties melted like butter (we discovered in fact that this tended to happen to objections whenever the objectors and Mrs. Wilholm met in person!). Regulations got bent and we had the sardonic satisfaction of seeing other people trying to wring blood out of a stone on Mrs. Wilholm's behalf. But to no avail—we had to transfer our whole apparatus, lock stock and barrel (the purchase of the block and tackle initially came out of a small fund built up from lecture fees and donations that the Team receive from time to time. Later, when some members of the Management Committee saw the film of events, the money was repaid into the Fund).

There were many alarms and excursions and many clashes with all sorts of strange forms of bureaucracy. One of the strangest was over her bath. We had noticed that all the old baths were being taken out of the flats and newer models installed. As Mrs. Wilholm had not used hers for many years and was unlikely to need it again, but did need the space it took up in her kitchen, we asked if her old one could be removed and no replacement made. This was ruled not to be possible as the next occupant of the flat might need one. In the end, no action was taken whatsoever—neither old one out nor new one in! Eventually, on 'D' Day minus one, our engineers, in their own time, went to her house and erected the hoist. So enthusiastic had they become that they had already painted it and an old iron hospital bedstead to which it was fixed so that it fitted in with her decor. The *piece de resistance* was the fact that they took along a small tin of paint to the house to touch up any marks they made when reassembling the hoist.

Her daughter went home to clean through and have things ready and was there early to meet Mrs. Wilholm on 'D' Day. In the late afternoon of 'D' Day the physiotherapist and doctor called to make sure all was well and watch a trial run of the hoist, and to make sure that the patient could get to the kitchen and turn on and off the lights. She already had an arrangement with a friend across the road that if she saw a little light in the window, help was needed. (The GPO had not yet found it possible to install a telephone). All seemed serene. It was a Friday. When the daughter called on Sunday, she found Mrs. Wilholm gaily cooking her Sunday joint, having re-cleaned all the brass ornaments 'properly', poor daughter having done them earlier in the week. When we next called, Mrs. Wilholm had also dealt with the one problem we had overlooked—namely, how to pull the curtains over her high windows. She had got her son-in-law and grandsons to lift the wheel-chair over the lintel and they had taken her to Woolworth's (she had not been to the shops for seven years) and she had bought some curtain cords and got them to fix these for her.

The next alarm was a week later when there was a call from the family doctor who had been kept well in the picture by telephone and letter. Mrs. Wilholm's bowels had failed to act. Reassurance was offered to him that she had gone up to three weeks on the ward without too dire results. After two weeks we hastily popped in to review her general condition, which we found to be good, and we relaxed again, despite the continuing bowel inaction. On the twenty-fifth day the telephone was installed and we rang Mrs. Wilholm to mark the occasion. On learning that the bowel inaction continued, readmission was offered for a day or two in order to effect dis-impaction. Mrs. Wilholm refused. Next day, Mafeking was reported to be relieved. Mrs. Wilholm told us later that she took a bottle of Eno's, a small bottle of Petrolagar, a whole packet of Ex-lax tablets and six Senokot tablets. As she said, rather than return to hospital, she felt drastic treatment was needed.

The home nurse was a brick, once she had recovered from the fact that the bed was fixed against the wall and window sill and could not be made in correct fashion. This was by design and necessity, so that Mrs. Wilholm could roll herself over in safety, but it was one handicap we had discussed. However, Mrs. Wilholm's daughter had been quite happy to make the bed once a week by climbing up on to it; in any case, as she pointed out, not many people do a thorough hospital bed-making job daily and Mrs. Wilholm said she was a very tidy sleeper.

So life slipped back into normal pattern and probably Mrs. Wilholm had more visitors than she had ever had in her life. The home nurse only needed to go twice a week but went daily. The home help went more frequently than she need, a chain of voluntary workers from the church did shopping and the welfare officer confessed that whenever she was visiting in that area her car's nose seemed inevitably to point in Mrs. Wilholm's direction.

She was home for two months and on the return of most of the Team from summer holidays, it was heard that she was ill in bed at home, vomiting and with a temperature. Not too much anxiety was felt as these symptoms had occurred before. She had had several urinary infections and it was known that a hiatus hernia, dealt with surgically about fifteen years before, had been shown radiologically to have recurred. Further extensive investigations had failed to reveal, when she was in hospital, any other cause for the temperatures or the vomiting or the severe pain she used to have in her back. In all conscience, she had enough skeletal disease to account for almost anything.

The hospital physician who knew her best revisited and found her very low, lying miserably in bed in a darkened room. Her daughter, who by now had great confidence in the hospital and knew that action would be taken if needed, was sitting placidly knitting by her side, trying to comfort her. With great delicacy, the question of readmission was raised and Mrs. Wilholm agreed—a very significant omen.

Soon after her return to hospital she had such a massive haemorrhage from her bladder that she required a blood transfusion. A special X-ray revealed the unhappy fact that she had a large cancer of the bladder. The genito-urinary surgeon did not feel even an examination under anaesthesia was necessary but such was Mrs. Wilholm's insistence, we had to use all our combined persuasive power to get a cystoscopy and biopsy done. It was such a huge growth that there was no hope of surgery nor really of radiation but we asked the radiotherapy consultant to see her just in case.

He wrote his opinion on the notes, that nothing was possible, and we increased the strength of the sedative drugs. They did not help and Mrs. Wilholm was inconsolable. Again time passed before we realised that she had been awaiting the result of the second expert's opinion and she had not seen the second consultant. He had read the reports and seen the X-rays in the ward's office, had written his views, but had never actually met Mrs. Wilholm. Her family had been told the verdict and they, like we, wished Mrs. Wilholm to pass painlessly away. She was then having injections three-hourly to dull the pain as she could keep little down by mouth. Soon, the nurses were in difficulty; she was watching the clock and clamouring for her injection on the dot, and even when the dose was doubled it did not seem to help.

The doctors had an anxious conclave. One who had considerable experience of the patient was unhappy with the situation, finding it impossible to maintain a relationship, which was longstanding, without telling the truth. Another felt it was unkind to give the stark truth in the patient's last days. A third, with some psychiatric experience but not knowing the patient, put forward a view that this was not an unknown phenomenon. The patient, who had no idea of the purpose of the injections, would presume they were given in order to cure, but if she knew they were making her no better, only by continually drawing the doctors' attention to the fact that they were doing no good, would she stimulate them into action. If she were told the truth, then she might find it easier.

This advice was followed. Mrs. Wilholm asked if no action was possible. She was willing to undergo any manner of surgery or X-ray treatment, but when she was assured that medical science had shot its bolt, she said quietly, "It's up to me then?" When this was agreed, she said, "Right, I will just have to make the best of it". And this is just what she did. From that point on, she needed no more sedation than an occasional dose of paracetamol, for she refused injections or stronger analgesics; she was much more tranquil and more her cheerful self again. She extracted a promise from the ward sister that her bed should not be moved from the centre of the ward to the side-room where most people were moved when they were dying, in order that they should not be disturbed by the noise in the main ward. Ten days later she slipped gracefully into death, closing a very momentous chapter. An autopsy revealed ten pathological conditions, any one of which could, in itself, have caused her death.

So very much was learnt from Mrs. Wilholm about people and things and procedures. So much was called for from each discipline and each discipline needed to have had so much hard basic training and experience in order to play an adequate part in her drama.

Once again it was proven that the actual disease processes were of the least significance where the patient's desire for independence and her spontaneous drive towards it was of all pervading importance. If the cancer had been discovered earlier, it would have made no difference to treatment prospects, but it would have meant that little effort would have been made to get Mrs. Wilholm home and she would have dwindled drearily away. Alternatively, it is often suggested that when there are so many people in need and so few staff available, we should give thinner slices of cake to more people instead of using such concentrated efforts on a few. This is, in fact, only a theoretical possibility. Some people are examples of the 'all or none' law. If Mrs. Wilholm could not have gone home and we had made no effort (disregarding the cancer for the moment), she would, literally and metaphorically, have turned her face to the wall, as she once did, but she would not necessarily have died. She could have gone on resentfully and despondently occupying a long-stay bed for another ten to twenty years. This has happened before now, and not infrequently.

From our experience, there is little doubt that when people are working under pressure, a natural order of priorities seems to emerge. Some, apparently, very unprepossessing people, one recognises instinctively as having potential towards personal independence and they need to be worked with, *despite themselves*; others, by their own spontaneity and very personalities, produce from the people around them the activity and support they need to help them.

Looking back upon Mrs. Wilholm's story, many things stand out, but three above all others :

1) Structural disease is not the most important thing : function is what counts.
2) An indomitable personality can, with support, overcome the most awe-inspiring disability.
3) None of the professional disciplines used in Mrs. Wilholm's support had really played their parts according to the book, in the way they had been trained. No formal training or text book could possibly have covered Mrs. Wilholm's needs. Even the nurses found that she called for more unorthodox treatment than most patients.

"Ah, but a man's reach should exceed his grasp,
or what's a heaven for?"

Browning

Chapter Seven

THE WAITING GAME

"The technical treatment of disease processes alone is quite inadequate".[1]

It was a general medical emergency this time—a patient who had been admitted to one of Dr. Binks' general medical beds—'acute', if one uses this term. *MRS. COCHRANE* was aged 82 and filthy dirty, with the dirt that one only finds in long-standing self-neglect. She had had a stroke and, as she lived alone, had lain on the floor for many hours before she was found. In Mrs. Cochrane's characteristic manner, she attributed her 'dishevelment' to having lain on the floor so long—a splendidly proud woman.

She had a right hemiplegia and speech difficulty and her general condition was so poor that she developed pressure sores rapidly. A naturally strong constitution and very good nursing support, with a minimum of drugs, won the day, and she began to regain strength. The main drawback was a deep pressure sore on her heel which also was characteristic of its kind, and because of the poor circulation to this area, quick to happen but very slow to heal.

Mrs. Cochrane herself was a tremendous personality who never looked her chronological age even in her bleakest hours. She always sat very erect and was always willing to declaim on any subject. She had natural theatrical talents and had produced many shows for her various social clubs; had made all the costumes, designed the sets, arranged the choreography and played the piano to boot. She revealed that she had done her last show only five months previously, and though it seemed hard to believe this, it was confirmed.

The speech therapist saw her (or perhaps one should say

Mrs. Cochrane was delighted to receive the speech therapist) and had helped greatly, for Mrs. Cochrane was very conscious of her dysphasia and developed a habit of putting her hand up to her mouth when speaking, as though to cover the defective words. They also began to practise left-handed writing together, just in case use did not return to the right hand, for, as in so many cases of speech difficulty, communication, whatever form it should take, is of paramount importance.

The occupational therapists were instant successes, as Mrs. Cochrane was a keen handicraft worker, and the group classes in the ward were meat and drink to her. She was soon the forewoman of her group, organising and enlivening whatever project happened to be in hand. She never needed to be reminded to bring her right hand into everything as she so much wanted to play the piano again. There was some slight embarrassment here, for the clothes she had worn on admission had had to be cut off her and destroyed, and we like our patients to be dressed in their own clothes and to be as normal as possible within the constraints of the inadequate ward environment (we have some wardrobe lockers but there is no storage space for clothes). She got a neighbour to bring things in. There was no doubt that her clothes were very tatty and moth eaten, but Mrs. Cochrane carried this off and one found that various members of the staff, from time to time, discreetly transfused her meagre supply of garments. Very, very, discreetly was this done, for Mrs. Cochrane was indeed a very proud woman.

When the heel had almost healed and she, with her walking frame, was independent, she went up to Springbok House 'to harden off' before going home, for to go home was her full intention and she would not sell her house, in which she was so lonely and which was such a headache to her. No. She had lived there forty years or more; she and her husband had moved there when it was in the country and there she would remain. Whilst in hospital she had obtained new dentures and glasses, had had chiropody and had seen about her hearing aid, so she felt happier about facing the world again.

At Springbok House life began to regain some savour. She was able to refurbish her wardrobe from the 'clothing shop', this being a master stroke of matron's and the voluntary workers' who helped there. Early on, Springbok House had acquired a supply of good second-hand clothing, so that residents with inadequate supplies could be helped; but it always proved difficult to effect, for inevitably people were very sensitive about accepting cast-off clothing, however good or however clean. Once a week a stall was set up in the hall with a suit, dress and coat rack by it and a variety of clothes put out for inspection and sale. This has completely altered the sartorial standard of Springbok—a dress for 10d. or a suit for 2s. is a bargain—before, it was charity. The original idea was to obtain a float of money and so buy in a stock of new things, such as new underwear and stockings, but the first consignment hung fire for so long, it was never tried again. The prices were inevitably beyond the 16s. a week pocket money—the average income of a person who has been in the hospital for a certain length of time.

So Mrs. Cochrane became much smarter and her hand improved to such an extent that two months later she was very shyly, and when everyone else had gone to bed, trying herself out on the piano. It was a success. She was still 'just going home' and dodged any attempts to hold realistic conversations on the subject. She had to have some more dental treatment about then, as there were some loose tooth fragments that had to be excised from her jaw. She reacted so violently to this suggestion and became so enraged, that we had to discontinue engagements with the Dental Department for a time. Plainly, she was undergoing considerable mental trauma about the future, but she continued to bury her head deep in the sand; it would be all right—she had friends and neighbours—when she got home she would sort it all out. Why were we not sending her home?

After the medical social worker had negotiated with Mrs. Cochrane's good next door neighbours about it, Mrs. Cochrane went home for a week-end's trial. Neighbours reported it as being unsuccessful as Mrs. Cochrane expected them to do everything for her and summoned them continually, this being possible by an intercommunicating bell they had installed for her. They also mentioned for the first time that the house had only gas lighting and paraffin heating. Mrs. Cochrane's report on the week-end was, of course, entirely different. Everything had gone like clockwork.

There was then a breathing space; she had an abscess round her dental stump and she eventually asked to have help from the Dental Department again. Meanwhile, her family doctor had got in touch with us, very disturbed at the prospect of Mrs. Cochrane's return home; he did not feel this to be at all rational.

We then decided that one or more of our team should go home with Mrs. Cochrane next time she went and so evaluate what was wanted and how much help and adaptation she would need. A keen young occupational therapist who had formed a very good relationship with Mrs. Cochrane and one of our new reablists who also happened to have a car took her home. They returned very shaken and upset, neither of them having made a visit of this nature before.

They reported the house to be a death trap, full of paraffin stoves and oil lamps, packed with furniture and every square inch otherwise crammed or lined with paper of one sort or another. Paper pictures, frills and decorations were stuck gaily all over the walls and every paper costume that Mrs. Cochrane had ever made for her shows was stored in her unused rooms, spilling over floor and furniture upstairs and downstairs. Apart from this, neglect was rampant in all its most depressing forms. Poor Mrs. Cochrane had been very nervous on the way home and most apologetic on arrival, commenting accurately that things had got very untidy in her absence, but it must have helped her to some realism, seeing her home afresh through the eyes of her new friends. She spontaneously considered that she would have to get rid of some of her furniture; she had four sofas in two very small rooms, and several suites of chairs, and thought these could be reduced in number.

Next time we talked of her discharge together, she was told firmly that this could not be with medical consent until some drastic action had been taken about her form of heating, lighting and cooking. The possibility of stumbling, even with her faithful walking frame, and knocking over one of her paraffin appliances, was too real in her Aladdin's cave of paper treasure. This brought a response from Mrs. Cochrane at once, via her pride. Her brother had often offered to electrify the house for her, but she had refused because she wished to be independent. The wedge was inserted into the crack with the speed of a rock climber on a tricky wall face and we hung on to it.

Her brother, a widower and wealthy, was only too delighted to be able to help his older sister at long last. The first necessity was to muster help to clear out the top layer of rubbish so that there would be enough visibility for estimates to be given for the work. With Mrs. Cochrane's consent and instruction, this was done. The paraffin galaxy was disposed of and gas fires installed in the two downstairs rooms used by Mrs. Cochrane. A new gas stove was put in the kitchen (the other one must surely have been one of the first models invented), a gas water heater installed over the sink, the whole ground floor wired for electricity and wall-to-wall carpeting laid in the two rooms and passages. Before this was done, a social task force from a nearby public school stripped, cleaned and re-papered and painted the rooms and kitchen in a colour scheme chosen and approved by Mrs. Cochrane. She would only allow the lower half of the house to be re-wired as she said she would never be going upstairs again and she had no intention of ever using it. She already had a downstairs w.c., so there was no problem here.

All these arrangements took time and there were many crises of one sort or another. The brother was burgled at his home on the East Coast and was too shocked to travel and supervise arrangements for a prolonged period. School holidays were needed for the task force. Electricity and Gas Company problems need no relating. The first fires installed had controls at the bottom and these had to be changed to ones with controls at the top. Meanwhile, Mrs. Cochrane fretted and fumed and had one ache, pain and physical complaint after another; but suddenly she ceased to complain and was always smiling, content and benevolent. At the same period another of the patients—a man who was also at Springbok House awaiting admission to a local authority residential home, ceased to complain and to moan. The staff reported that the couple were always together and we took it lightly, but one day they announced their engagement. It was no longer a joke, for we had known the man for many years and knew that Mrs. Cochrane could never hope to cope with him. Apart from his temperament, his physical disabilities, which were unknown to her, were far too great for an even older, and herself a handicapped person, to deal with on a long-term basis.

This was a doctor's dilemma. It would have been a breach of professional confidence to tell Mrs. Cochrane why it was not advisable. There was nothing to do but grin, bear it and pray that merciful providence would intervene in some way. Mrs. Cochrane intended a wedding before she left Springbok House and told matron that she could have the honour of catering for the reception. It was felt that the only hope was somehow to get Mrs. Cochrane home first and then her own good sense might come to the rescue. The doctor desperately advocated not marrying, but just living on a friendly trial basis at first but this really upset Mrs. Cochrane's sense of propriety—she could not possibly share a bed with a man unless they were married. They were actually contemplating disposing of her single beds and obtaining a double one! There was nothing left but hope.

Mrs. Cochrane kept making forays down to her house by day and also over-night trips, preparing things. Her brother became anxious—all was now complete—was she ever moving back again? As by this time she had been with us for twenty-two months, we felt it was important not to spoil the ship for a ha'porth of tar and we held the line. Christmas came; the cold weather came; she would "decide next week"; "traffic will be difficult". Then suddenly she announced her departure for two days ahead. The entry in her notes says, somewhat cynically, "Says she's going home permanently on Wednesday—there is bound to be a snowstorm that day".

There was no snowstorm. She went. We decided against follow-up clinic appointments, but arranged with her family doctor that our team would occasionally drop in and see her when passing. We tried to arrange for her to attend the Work Centre which was just nearby her home and which we thought would give her a focus, and distract her mind from her fiance, who had suddenly developed a profound anaemia and had had to be readmitted to the ward for further investigation. Mrs. Cochrane was charming but firm—she would go to the centre when she had tidied things up at home—there were many things she had to do first and it would more than fill her days.

We despaired, for we saw her reverting to her old rut. The next time the hospital doctor called in to see her at home she had called in a carpenter and a new second hand-rail had been fitted to the wall on the stairs. Why? Mrs. Cochrane had promised not to bother with upstairs. She explained patiently that she had to clear up the mess there first, and whilst the subject was under discussion, could she have a second walking frame—she would need to have one upstairs and one down. And did the doctor like this beautiful electric light shade she had designed and made in readiness whilst at Springbok House? Oh, and wouldn't the doctor like to see her garden? This turned out to be a typical piece of Mrs. Cochrane's whimsical humour. She had a window box outside her window and had carefully planted it with a 'garden' full of plastic flowers.

On another visit Mrs. Cochrane was upstairs, plus her walking frame, with a young boy scout whom she had commandeered to help her burn old mattresses and paper costumes, etc. Each time, she enquired tenderly after her fiance who she knew by this time was mortally ill, but she managed to visit him with the help of friends with cars.

Her family doctor rang again; a new home nurse, whilst helping to blanket bath her, had discovered a lump in her breast. The query now was what to do. We agreed on hormone treatment but the family doctor would be grateful if the hospital physician would visit first; this was agreed and a date decided upon. Just before leaving to visit, the news came from the ward of her fiance's death. By the time the physician got to Mrs. Cochrane she too knew—the man's relatives, who had adopted her as part of the family, having let her know at once. She was very philosophical—she knew it had to come—and then she got down to the subject of her own lump. She wanted neither surgery nor radiotherapy, please, and was happy to settle for pills. Had she thought any more about the Work Centre? Yes, but she had too much to do at home still. The doctor wearily registered yet one more polite brush-off. As though sensing the disappointment, Mrs. Cochrane proudly displayed some old chairs she had had re-covered and done up most charmingly. There was no doubt about it, she really was doing what she had said she was going to do.

A month or two passed and we heard that she was going to the Work Centre five afternoons a week and was as happy as a sand-boy, and, of course, was one of the best workers. To start a new life and go back to work again at 85 is not bad going, especially when one remembers Mrs. Cochrane's condition and social circumstances three years before.

This is a success story. I think it would be impossible to doubt this fact. Related on paper, it looks sensible, reasonable and the only way in which the situation could have been managed. It would be an injustice, however, to let the case rest there, for without there being integrity of purpose, a master plan and a true willingness from top to bottom to give appropriate support to Mrs. Cochrane until she found a satisfactory way of living, this result could never have been achieved. Even in her case there were murmurings from time to time that she should not be permitted to go on 'blocking' a bed; she should be told what she should do and how and when, and anyway, she should be made to give up her home and go into an Old People's Home and be looked after properly. At every stage, without free communication between the team involved, and a common purpose, the delicate ship might have been capsized.

Mrs. Cochrane's story makes the point better than most, that the policy of having 'acute' and 'chronic' geriatric wards is a dangerous one. In some hospitals it is the policy to banish patients who do not 'make the grade' in six months to chronic wards where they receive custodial care. One has heard that in some places such failures may not even be reviewed medically again except for certification purposes. Let us make sure that such places become extinct very soon.

On the other hand, suppose we had acceded to this prevailing sense of alarm and urgency that infiltrates everywhere that there is a huge queue of potential patients lining up outside our hospital doors, clamouring to be admitted or they will perish. We know, for instance, that in our own particular area—North West Middlesex—there are 750 more 'acute' hospital beds than are considered needful for the population at risk. There is a deficiency of 270 geriatric beds by the same national standards. Convert some of the surplus 'acute' into 'geriatric' and we are still left with 480 surplus to the accepted need. It does not seem rational, therefore, that anyone should perish from lack of a bed in a hospital.

It is also known that many so-called 'acute' hospitals are running 60 to 70 per cent bed occupancy. Our beds have a 97 per cent bed occupancy, and this, despite the fact that we are constantly being unable to use beds because of lack of staff.

If Mrs. Cochrane had been forced to acquiesce to a "tidy, short-cut solution"—to give up her home and go into a residential Home, would her very real but intangible needs as an individual have been fulfilled? In all probability she would have deteriorated both physically and mentally, as she often did with us when things were not shaping well towards her ends, and then she would have returned to us very soon.

Historically, in our own department, in an attempt to overcome the shortage of geriatric beds, the system of 'rationing' was introduced. As many people as possible were given a period of six weeks in hospital and 'intensive treatment' was applied. This resulted in a waiting list of 350 because of the high relapse rate and because a promise of readmission had to be given to relatives in many instances, as might be expected when people in need of hospital support were being returned home. In time, the system defeated itself because it became impractical to honour the undertakings.

It is the firm belief of this particular Geriatric Department that spending more time at the outset saves time in the long run, besides reducing individual human suffering and discomfort. This, Mrs. Cochrane's story illustrates so well.

> "My pride struck out new sparkles of her
> own. Such was I, such by nature still
> I am".
>
> *John Dryden*

Reference

1. Binks, F. Allen. (1968). *Brit. Med. J.*, **i**, 269-74.

Chapter Eight

DEFEAT

"Admission to hospital is needed when the home is not a true home and medical and nursing help is needed in an emergency which cannot be provided effectively in any other way".[1]

One of the most stimulating things about domiciliary visiting is that one can never tell from letters, messages or even by direct contact with the family doctor just what situation one is going to meet until one actually visits.

A classic example of this occurred one October when the department was working without one of the senior doctors and no houseman. Requests for help were flooding in and the doctor dealing with the message book found one morning a request telephoned by a doctor's secretary which stated: "Request for outpatient clinic appointment—a sitting case with husband as escort—on expectorants and sedatives—? what. Motor neurone disease. We are being asked to see patient with a view to terminal care".

At this point our secretary had obviously demurred at the incongruity and the family doctor himself had taken over the telephone and said an early appointment must be given as the patient had difficulty in swallowing. She was not incontinent and had been under the care of another physician at the hospital in the past.

We retrieved the old hospital records and found that she had been seen in the Out-Patient Clinic of another physician, some months previously, and in his letter the consultant had specifically asked for a re-referral if the GP was not happy about things.

The next move, patently, was to telephone the family doctor

and find out why we were needed. This was done and a most surprising conversation ensued. The patient, *MRS. CONSTANT* was said to be dying and in need of urgent admission : if no admission possible at once, could she be visited urgently? After the preliminary skirmish, the history was given of the intervening months.

Instead of sending her back to my colleague when she had not improved, she had been sent to the specialist neurological hospital in Town. She was diagnosed there as having cerebrovascular degeneration of the pons and she and her husband were told there was nothing that could be done about it. The hospital then wrote to the family doctor who tried to explain to the husband that it was a lethal condition; no treatment was possible and she would die of starvation as her powers of swallowing would go altogether in time.

This had all occurred one year before the request to us for help, and the family reported that the prognosis was now being fulfilled. It was suggested to the family doctor that if the patient was reasonably fit, there were still certain surgical procedures possible and why not refer back to the specialist hospital where more help of this type would be available? He said that they did not seem to want to know about Mrs. Constant any more and he was at his wits' end. He would refer her wherever it was suggested if we wished—this after mentioning hospitals for the dying—but he never had success in that direction. The whole situation seemed so desperate, and the GP so negative, that a domiciliary visit seemed the only thing to do. There was the possibility of a vacancy on one of the women's wards, and it was necessary to establish which of several patients had the greatest need of hospital admission.

The visiting physician located the block of old people's flats off the main road. The Constants, both aged 71, lived in a first-floor flat. A small, wiry, thin woman with a welcoming smile opened the door and indicated that she was Mrs. Constant. She was fully dressed. She led the doctor into her rather depressing sitting-room where sat, slumped on an even more depressed sofa, an unshaven, bronchitic, wheezing, saturnine little man and another elderly woman (her sister)—deaf but very friendly and with a bracing air about her.

There was an atmosphere of tension in the room and it soon became clear why. Mrs. Constant given time, patience and a relaxed atmosphere could still speak a little and make herself understood but her husband spoke for her or else contradicted everything she tried to say. At frequent intervals he pointed out that his wife was done for—how could a man be cheerful when, after fifty years of marriage, his wife was going to die and leave him alone, with no one to look after him? Of course, she could not eat or do anything; she was starving to death and it was not fair.

All attempts to explain about semi-solid food, such as jellies, junkets or porridge, etc., being best fell on deaf ears. If she was not able to eat the things he bought for them, such as pie and meat, then that was that. The doctor looked hopefully at the sister—could she not invite Mrs. Constant to her house for a meal occasionally? The change would do her good. She agreed but looked dolefully at the husband who refused to let Mrs. Constant go anywhere without him "in case she collapsed".

Mrs. Constant did not want to go into hospital and had no such need at that time, but she agreed to attend the out-patient clinic. The doctor made a note on the visit report that although the patient *had* plenty of pathology, there was no need to be thinking in terms of terminal care; the main trouble was the husband's attitude. Mrs. Constant's greatest need was obviously to be able to go away from her husband for a time and his devastating, undermining influence. She had a delightful sense of humour, and life must be like living in a black cloud for her. Another suggestion was that Mrs. Constant would be a good candidate for a combined team 'think' in the FAC which was soon to be opened.

A daughter came with Mrs. Constant to the first out-patient appointment and provided a good deal of information about Mr. Constant. She said that the flat was scheduled for repairs and redecoration but he refused to have anything done as they would not be there much longer. There were two daughters, and Mrs. Constant had several sisters. All the family would do anything in the world for Mrs. Constant and have her to stay with them any time but as Mr. Constant refused to let her go away without him and no one would have him to stay, their efforts were frustrated.

The routine clinical investigations were done and a combined assault was mustered. The speech therapist devised various trick movements and exercises to see if she could help Mrs. Constant's swallowing capabilities. The dietician worked out suitable menus and the occupational therapist and physiotherapist worked out ways and means of helping the residual right-sided weakness. The most important thing of all—the medical social workers started getting to know Mr. Constant for we all felt that although, indeed, Mrs. Constant needed much physical help to make life as satisfactory as possible until the inexorable end arrived, it would still be a year or more away, and if Mr. Constant's attitude could be softened, perhaps things would be more tolerable for her.

Amongst ourselves we expressed our opinions of hospitals which created situations and then failed to accept responsibility.

[We still have in one of our annexes a delightful lady who had attended a teaching hospital for ten years with high blood pressure. They showed great interest in her—she was often asked to come in for a week whilst examinations were on, to be 'clinical material'. She had had several minor strokes and had become slightly more handicapped. On one of her regular visits a consultant drew the husband aside and said solemnly, "All that can be done has been done and her life is now drawing to a close. We can do no more for her and she has no need to attend hospital further". The family were heartbroken. The only daughter and her husband gave up their home and moved in with the old couple. The old lady's husband gave up his job and they devoted themselves to making the patient's last year happy. Two years later the family were exhausted and the patient fat and almost atrophied from lack of exercise. We were asked to help because the husband was being investigated for symptoms he had ignored for two years in order to look after his wife. They both came into hospital. She was soon skipping about like a spring lamb and he had had an abdomino-perineal resection for cancer of the rectum. They returned home. She deteriorated again because the family could not break the habit of over-solicitude. She came in and out three times in all—then he died and she had another stroke and is still fatly with us—ten years after "no more could be done for her".]

And this was Mrs. Constant's problem. Indeed no more

could be done for her as far as technical scientific medicine was concerned but this did not mean that she promptly ceased to exist. This surely was just the time when she and her family needed the most support available, for to be written off, and yet not be dead, must be the most terrifying experience known. Strangely enough, she was not even given the *coup de grace*—a course of physiotherapy! The feature that is always particularly galling and which also tends to nullify one's efforts to help, as in Mrs. Constant's case, is that the specialist hospital, with all its resources, has the reputation of Mecca whereas the local district hospital, with its inadequate staffing facility ratio, has little glamour, particularly as it has to cope with the rejects of the selective system—the really tough problems, such as Mrs. Constant and the lady whose life was "drawing to a close". Mr. Constant said repeatedly—what was the use of all the things we were doing or suggesting when the specialist hospital had said that nothing could be done and his own GP had repeated it and confirmed it by rarely coming to see her? Why were we busying ourselves in this manner? We should let her die in peace.

It was futile to keep pointing out to Mr. Constant that on the contrary, Mrs. Constant was very much alive and kicking and wanting to live. She was then coming up to the OT Department three times a week and having a specially prepared lunch, quietly by herself, taking her time over it. The food was so highly concentrated with calories and proteins that one felt mildly surprised that it did not propel itself into Mrs. Constant's mouth! But it was working and she was gaining a little weight. We would have liked her to come five days a week but she had chores to do on the other days, one of which was to draw her own pension which she handled herself—a source of constant annoyance to Mr. Constant, who had retired at the first opportunity available and never done anything further although he was a barber and could easily have made more pocket money for himself. In fact, it was a bait we tried, to distract his attention from his wife. We thought that a small part-time barbering job, with transport provided, would please him, but no, he preferred National Assistance.

Mrs. Constant also did small jobs in the OT Department. She tended the indoor plants, of which there is a profusion, and helped less mobile patients with their work. She continued her speech therapy sessions and once a week she went over to the ward and had a bath. She had shyly written a note, to ask if there was any possibility of this, as she found getting in and out of a bath a great difficulty and her husband made such a fuss if she asked him to help. Obviously, he considered, a dying woman should not be needing a bath! Another of Mrs. Constant's problems was sleeping. They had a double bed and Mr. Constant complained bitterly that she kept him awake all night. Single beds were suggested but Mr. Constant would have none of this as he said she needed his help when she woke with her coughing! More often than not, Mrs. Constant would remain all night in the sitting room, miserably curled up on the sofa.

Time after time she was seen in the clinic and her husband always came and belligerently denied any improvement, although this palpably had occurred, in her general condition. Several social workers broke on the rock of Mr. Constant. An ex-geriatric nurse from the North came to live near with her husband and new baby. She approached us, asking if anyone within walking distance needed visiting—she would like to help if she could. Manna from Heaven it seemed to us—someone with inside knowledge, but living near, who could take a personal interest and perhaps help Mrs. Constant with the preparation of suitable meals. She was thoroughly briefed and trudged round, with the baby in the pram—a less official looking person there never was.

Meanwhile, there was a slight thaw. The social worker had got Mr. Constant to agree to let his wife go away to the seaside with a party going from the borough. At the same time arrangements were made for her to attend a club near home. She was physically in much better shape and now weighed as much as she had ever done in her life, except when she had been pregnant.

She went on the holiday, with tremendous anticipation, but after a week wrote pitifully asking to be brought back. Firstly, she had been put in a room with another woman who smoked incessantly, which nearly choked Mrs. Constant, and then she had heard some of the helpers referring to her as "a dumbie who was cracked in the head". This, with the unpalatable food, was too much for even Mrs. Constant's *joie de vivre*. Mr. Constant was triumphant and gloated greatly over this, and from then on redoubled his efforts to stop her attending the OT Department. He frequently sent transport away, saying that Mrs. Constant was too ill. This manoeuvre was countered by a quick visit by a doctor and social worker to enquire blandly after Mrs. Constant's health; on discovering her sitting fully dressed and disconsolate because transport had failed to come for her (as she thought), the doctor and social worker gave her a lift to the hospital.

By now, Mrs. Constant's morale was beginning to crack and she developed a bad cold which slowly became a chest infection. We visited her again and tried to talk to her. All the time Mr. Constant's voice beat on relentlessly. We tried to distract him by discussing the World Cup Series which was then working up to its exciting climax, near to where they lived—but how could we expect a man to enjoy television when his wife could not even get up and cook a meal for him? The flat itself was much more cheerful, at least, for at last he had allowed the repairs and redecorations to be done. Mrs. Constant came into hospital and stayed precisely two weeks; she then felt well enough to go home. Perhaps, too, she was embarrassed, for her husband came daily and sat by her bed complaining and bemoaning his fate for all and sundry to hear—and Mrs. Constant was a proud woman.

The friendly nurse with the baby redoubled her efforts but was not allowed to prepare any meals or even a protein drink. Things were complicated too because even the baby took a dislike to Mr. Constant and screamed whenever he saw him, which meant that the baby had to be left outside the flats. At this juncture Mr. Constant talked incessantly about committing suicide when his wife died and this seemed a useful stage at which to ask the mental welfare authorities to help. Once more the hospital team went forth and met the mental welfare officer at the flat; arrangements having been made for Mrs. Constant to return to hospital, thus leaving the mental welfare officer to talk to Mr. Constant, and lay the foundation for his future support.

Mrs. Constant had much earlier on refused to consider surgical help so that food could be passed directly into her stomach, and one imagines that such a procedure would have been anathema to her very fastidious mind. She was happy to be among friends but obviously was thinking wistfully of home all the time, but her home did not quite add up to the definition of a true home—"a place where reasonable creature comforts exist (e.g. shelter, food, heat, light and simple sanitary facilities) where, besides the person concerned, at least one other reasonably fit person with interests, goodwill and commonsense is present most of the time and where the services of an interested family doctor are available".[2] Mrs. Constant died two years and eight months after her condition was diagnosed as bulbar palsy and the husband had been told that nothing could be done for her. How do doctors who make these statements think that sentient people are going to pass the time away subsequently? Mrs. Constant was not a special and unique case: I can, of my own experience, cite many scores such as she.

"Some live dying : best to die living."
Edward J. Stieglitz

References

1. Binks, F. Allen. (1962). *Lancet,* **i,** 1083-86.
2. *Ibidem.*

Chapter Nine

DEGENERATIVE DISEASE

"Effective social services will only be established if they fit without conflict into a total pattern of help which people provide for themselves and each other".[1]

MRS. FEATHER was 73. She had worked in a big draper's in London and before retiring had held a responsible job. She had worked for the same firm for forty-three years and they were sorry to lose her. They were large contributors to the Drapers' Homes—a well organised plan of sheltered housing, where the progressive needs of residents can be met by flexible types of accommodation—and they offered her a cottage for her retirement. Mrs. Feather had never been a home-body although she had been left with a small son and daughter to look after when her husband deserted her. She much preferred her business life contacts and housework bored her. As she had been more or less lodging with her daughter, Mrs. Faithful and her family, for fifteen years before retirement, she thought she would continue to do so and she turned down the cottage. Mrs. Feather was very gay and sprightly and Mr. Faithful liked her; Mrs. Faithful's children were young and it all looked as though it would work out well. They moved to a different house in a dormitory urban area and Mrs. Feather had her church contacts and the shopping to do.

Then she started a tremor of Parkinsonism and her hands began to develop contractures; she became more nervous of going out alone and her orbit and outside contacts began to diminish. Other problems began to arise too as she had to share a bedroom with her grand-daughter who was now 16; not surprisingly there was a certain amount of difficulty for both parties.

In order to try and help her locomotor problems, her doctor

sent her to a Physical Therapy Clinic nearby where she had wax bath treatment for her hands and a splint was made to help prevent further contraction; but none of these measures seemed to help and her demands on her daughter became more persistent and constant.

During Mr. and Mrs. Faithful's summer holiday, Mrs. Feather's elder sister, a very vigorous down to earth 80-year-old, and her husband came to stay to keep an eye on Mrs. Feather and the two grand-children. They were shocked at the way in which Mrs. Feather was going on. The sister commented that Mrs. Feather was the youngest of a big family and she had always depended on other people to do things for her. They tackled the family doctor about getting something done and the Geriatric Department were asked to help.

The doctor from the department duly visited and found the decor of the house so pleasantly colourful that a mental note was made that the department's new cine camera would find an excellent background for some filming. After talking to and examining Mrs. Feather and putting her through her paces, this thought was more than confirmed—that with adequate stimulus, e.g. a fresh audience, there was very little that she could not do for herself. She had a most fascinating way of getting herself on and off the lavatory seat, by going into the lavatory backwards. Her method of going up and down a precipitous flight of stairs with a nasty twist at the top and the banisters boarded in was, for the observer, a hair-raising marvel.

Her personality was one of tremendous sociability and her whole *raison d'etre* seemed to be people. As long as she had people to talk to she was perfectly happy. Never had there been a woman more ideally suited to the rather stultifying atmosphere of the 'no activity' often to be found in residential homes. In fact, on closer acquaintance, it transpired that this was where Mrs. Feather wished to be but she did not want to hurt her daughter's feelings by suggesting it. With all the family out all day, she was bored and lonely. She wished heartily that she had accepted the offer of a cottage when she had retired and she would never have wanted for companionship. She had a theory that she could always go into a residential home—part of the Drapers' tripartite scheme (cottages, Home and Nursing Home) any time she liked. The subject was broached with her daughter (who had had similar thoughts but did not want to hurt her mother's feelings by being the first to suggest it!) in a session in the FAC, and Mrs. Feather was keen that plans should go ahead as fast as possible. In consequence of this, she became vastly more cheerful and active.

Whilst negotiations were going on, she was coming by ambulance to the OT Department twice a week (the nearby Workrooms were inaccessible to her without transport). She enjoyed every minute of her trips. She was one of the few patients who did not mind how circuitously the ambulance came or went or how long it took, as long as she had company. She was extremely popular with everyone she met. She did very little actual work unless watched closely and would have everyone waiting on her in a flash, but in general she was a different woman.

The medical social worker found that she had left it too late for the Drapers' scheme; progression had to be from cottage to the Home part; there was no direct admission to the Home and Mrs. Feather was certainly not up to living alone in a cottage, even with a good deal of help. So application was made for her to go on to the borough residential homes waiting list. Never had we fewer misgivings about making such a recommendation. Sometimes this suggestion has to be made because there is no available practical alternative—but Mrs. Feather would be square peg in square hole and we visualised her having fairly speedy admission as she was such a prepossessing person. As a precautionary measure, however, we kept her coming up to the OP follow-up clinic and OT sessions with an occasional booster in the FAC to ensure that she was maintaining her mobility. We rested, as we had been assured some six weeks after we had first seen her that she had been accepted on the Welfare Home waiting list for an early vacancy. A month later we see a comment in her clinic notes that the welfare officer has visited again and assured her of the first vacancy after Christmas.

Here once more we have to plead the difficulties of maintaining continuity, for having established a plan and put it into action and seen things through into the right channel of communication, immediacy tends to fade and other priority situations crowd in.

This is what happened to Mrs. Feather. The routine supporting programme ground on. Mrs. Feather and her daughter were such nice people they did not complain or press, and different people began to see Mrs. Feather at her attendances, not fully appreciating that she was awaiting a place in a Home.

Then a chain reaction took place, and like a slow fuse, it gradually smouldered along its length until it blew sky high, precisely at the time when those who knew most about Mrs. Feather were on holiday. It seemed that the prolonged waiting period undermined Mrs. Feather's morale. She became more demanding and aggressive and would hardly let her daughter out of her sight or do anything for herself whilst at home. Mrs. Faithful's son was about to get married and leave the family home. Mrs. Faithful's daughter was at a very difficult teenage stage—not aided by her lack of at least a bedroom to herself, and as so often happens also Mrs. Faithful was undergoing all the difficulties of the menopause. The strains became so unbearable that this normally most controlled and sane of women eventually broke; went and locked herself in a room and smashed all the bric-a-brac available. It did not give her any relief, she said, but just made her feel very guilty.

She went to her doctor who prescribed some tranquillisers and told her to return in two weeks' time. The calm recital of her next visit is worth recording. She went into the surgery and a different doctor was on duty. He did not look at her but told her to sit down and asked her if she was on pills? He then pointed to three different sized circles, drawn on his blotting pad, and asked her to point out the approximate size of the tablets she was taking and to give a description of their texture, colour and markings. After this he wrote out a new prescription and told her to return in two weeks. She has not been back, nor has she taken any more pills : she realised that she would have to fight this battle alone.

She was not completely alone as she had one friend—a very respected member of the Borough Council, who decided that it was time something was done and who rang both the Welfare Department and the family doctor. In consequence, one of our doctors and another welfare officer visited the patient again, strangely enough choosing the very same day. At that stage it certainly looked as though the patient should be admitted to hospital, her function having so deteriorated, and she was put on the waiting list. Before she could be admitted, the holiday-making staff (to whom she was well known) returned and eventually heard the news, and because of the long-standing relationship with the patient, visited her at home. Apart from stairs, it was possible to encourage Mrs. Feather to do everything she had done on the first visit a year before. Her daughter withdrew, overcome; she had no realisation that her mother's function and capabilities had remained so good. She had thought that as her mother had a disease that was reputed to progress remorselessly, she had succumbed in the natural order of things, and felt guilty that she had not been able to make her mother do more. The difficulty with stairs was understandable: Mrs. Feather had fallen at the twist at the top some time before and lost her nerve but with assistance round the bend, she was quite able to 'sit' her way down, step by step, and went up them very well.

A lengthy discussion ensued between the interested parties as to the next move. Mrs. Feather was assured that there was no reluctance to have her in hospital—it was doubt as to need that made the doctor hesitate. She, herself, was anxious to get into a Home and settle down permanently. She knew it was all becoming too much for her daughter and she was very perturbed herself.

A further film was made of her function for comparison with the one made the year before. The subject was re-opened with our welfare colleagues. It took much persuasion and several meetings before they were convinced that Mrs. Feather's first move was to a Home and not to a hospital, but after long consideration they agreed to give her a two week trial at a Home after Christmas. They required our solemn assurance that we would help if things went wrong and the daughter's assurance and understanding that the patient was only to be admitted for a two week trial period, and if this was successful, she would be returned home to await a permanent vacancy. To us this did not seem a very happy plan but they were the best terms we could arrange. We held our breath, not daring to interfere when she went in to the Home on trial, in case some incautious word should prejudice Mrs. Feather's situation in the Home and make her *persona non grata.*

Perhaps this was where we made our next mistake. Mrs. Feather was a success beyond one's wildest dreams—the matron and staff loved her and they were very upset that she could not stay. We were also upset, but by a little blackmail and sacrifice of a place 'owed' to us, as we had recently taken a resident into hospital, we managed to make it possible for her to stay.

She was seen there at a later date by one of our doctors who was visiting another resident, and danger signals were noted. She was sitting in the corner of the sitting room, feet on a footstool and legs very swollen. Patently, she was sitting doing nothing all day and people were fetching and carrying for her. The matron said she was a 'sweety' and people loved her and they loved waiting on her—"it was no trouble". The doctor warned Mrs. Feather that she must do more for herself and keep active and she smiled prettily and said how she missed her trips to the OT Department and hoped all her friends were well!

A month or two later, again when visiting someone else, Mrs. Feather was seen *en passant*. The story was slightly different. There had been one or two staff crises; it was the end of the winter; people were tired of fetching and carrying, and supporting Mrs. Feather was a little less rewarding. The staff wished she would do more for herself; she was taking advantage of their kindness. They wished they had known originally how much she was capable of doing herself. A month later came the expected call from the Matron—Mrs. Feather had deteriorated suddenly and rapidly in the course of three days (*sic*). It was thought that her spine had crumbled, and she could not even feed herself with a spoon.

There was no need to visit. We knew. In she came, curled up like a dormouse and very confused. She had been having a fair amount of sedation and this probably accounted for her confusion, plus a marked degree of constipation. We stopped the sleeping pills, got her bowels moving and gradually got her up again. It was too late—the situation was not reversible. She made some slight progress but there was obviously no return and Mrs. Feather herself had lost enthusiasm. She had come to know us and rely on us only too well and felt secure. It was useless to attempt to force an issue. She moved to one of our long-stay annexes and remained as charmingly cheerful and gregarious as ever. The only positive result of her stay in a Home was a 'boy friend'. During her period there, another lady with Parkinsonism had been admitted with her husband, as a therapeutic experiment, to give her husband some support. Unfortunately she had died in the Home and the widower had returned to his flat alone, but he had struck up a friendship with Mrs. Feather, and despite his 84 years and a mile walk from the bus stop, he trudges along to see her once a week. He says that it is good to have an objective for getting dressed and going out and it makes him feel that he is still of some use.

Mrs. Feather herself has more to interest her and more activity round her than ever she did in the Home. Her daughter is a changed woman and their relationship is back to where it was, for her daughter mentioned that during the black period of waiting she got to the point where she hated her mother with savage ferocity. It had seemed as though her life was being drained out of her by the insistent demands being made upon her. She hated herself for this and she knew it was unfair but the omnipresence of her mother, coupled with the worries over her children and her own physiological changes, had been unbearable. Now she has spasms of guilt because there does not seem to be anything to worry about! However, she is able with her husband to contribute a good deal of help to the overworked staff of the annexe.

MISS PHOENIX was only 59, when I first became responsible for her medical welfare. At that stage she was one of the few patients in one of our long-stay annexes who was bedfast and it seemed reasonable to me that *status quo* should not be disturbed. She had had Parkinsonism since the age of 19. This had been progressive and she was really disabled by it. Moreover, she had an un-united fracture of her femur. At that stage in my career, knowledge dunned into me during my formal medical education remained uppermost in my mind, and I had seen little reason to think otherwise. People who had degenerative conditions, such as atherosclerosis, rheumatoid arthritis, Parkinson's disease and multiple sclerosis, always and inevitably deteriorated with the passage of time. Miss Phoenix had reached this stage and my function was to support the nurses in supporting her terminal stage and make life as tolerable as possible. For myself, I did not find our relationship easy because the mere sight of a doctor always precipitated a demand for more and different pills and medicines.

Soon after we got to know one another, she collapsed one day and developed a high temperature and all sorts of bizarre symptoms for which no adequate clinical explanation was ever found. It entailed much to-ing and fro-ing by day and night, as she hovered betwixt life and death. Some of her relatives (she had many brothers and sisters who visited rarely) came, and they were not in favour of her being moved away from the security of the annexe for heroic investigations and possible treatment at the parent hospital. In her lucid moments, neither was Miss Phoenix. She was cheered by the promises of some of her relatives with cars, that when the fine weather came they would take her out for drives. I learned a little more of her previous history; there was some talk of a broken engagement. Miss Phoenix had always been at home with her parents. Her mother was still alive at that time but too frail to come to see Miss Phoenix. There had been some family row and Miss Phoenix seemed to have been involved in it. Prior to her admission to hospital in 1953 with a broken hip, she had not walked for years. She and her mother were then living with a sister and brother-in-law and their two children. She was treated surgically and apparently was remobilised to the stage of walking with a tripod, but when it had come to discharging her home, the family struck. The sister felt that she had borne the heat of the day long enough and that some of the other eight or nine kith and kin should take a turn. From the brief laconic notes available, the battle raged between authority and family. Very big guns were turned on the erring sister and her husband, without success. They were both out at work and could not cope. Miss Phoenix was then moved into a geriatric annexe bed on the strict understanding that it was only for six weeks (this was the era of the Department's trial of the six-weeks In-and-Out System). Possible readmission at some later date was promised. Again the sister refused. Even firmer measures were now taken—the discharge notice, date and time were given and the patient was packed into an ambulance and sent home. She was warned that she might be rejected; she was. The ambulance men failed to gain admission and she was returned to hospital. Shortly after that she fell once more and the pin from the previous operation slipped and had to be left *in situ* as she was not considered to be fit enough for its removal. She was left with a slipped pin and an un-united fracture of her femur. After various attempts at remobilising her, it was decided to call it a day. She found it more comfortable being in bed than sitting up and it seemed that reasonably this should be allowed. She could still be got on to a commode but that was the total sum of her activity.

It is difficult to discover retrospectively what her thoughts must have been when she was sent home and returned again. It is also difficult to picture what relationships would have been like in the home if the family's nerve had broken in response to the shock tactics and they had taken her in. One cannot visualise there being any peace or security in such a situation, for either patient or family, and one regrets that these primitive manoeuvres are still happening. Some of our authoritarian colleagues still try to force relatives to subjection by these punitive measures, failing to see that it can only exacerbate the situation that must have already gone beyond recall. Bad enough to do this with a patient who is reasonably independent for his personal needs, but whose temperament is incompatible. How indefensible to send home in this manner someone who still has a clear call on hospital support—for instance, a man, confused, incontinent and bedridden.

Not many months ago we were called by a medical officer of health (from whom the family doctor had asked for help) to see a man in his eighties sent home to a frail wife of similar age. The man was so confused, noisy and uncontrollable, apart from being doubly incontinent, that the hospital had also sent a cot-sided bed out with him. (Slight Freudian symbolism there—it was obviously realised that he still needed a hospital bed!). The rationale behind this action was that he had been admitted for treatment of a chest infection, which had been duly treated. In the process he had been kept in bed, given barbiturate sleeping tablets which had made him confused and increased his constipation, and he had become uraemic and totally unaware of what he was doing. He was then a disturbance to other patients in the ward and therefore had to go home. The doctor concerned felt free to do this because the patient had been treated and cured of the illness for which he had been admitted and the old wife was too conscientious to emulate Miss Phoenix's relatives and refuse to accept him.

Again, this is not a special or extreme case. It can be matched by instances that come to our knowledge day in and day out. The unscrupulous reasoning behind such action is an underlying form of blackmail. The Geriatric Department is known to have a collective conscience and a sense of area responsibility, and the suggestion is frequently made that if a patient is sent home in this way, the Geriatric Department will admit him within the following two weeks; but if he remains where he is, he will never get the specialised treatment he needs and which only the Geriatric Department can give because 'they' will not take over patients from other hospitals—"it is unethical". There is little doubt that the firm line being taken (mainly through force of circumstances of the too large area and too few beds) in recent years to try and encourage other departments to accept their own responsibilities for long-stay patients is producing a tremendous reaction of irresponsible aggression from our medical colleagues.

Shades of the Poor Law and the National Health Service Act of 1948. Doctors have not yet grasped that 'chronic hospitals' have ceased to exist and there are no longer human warehouses where 'clinical failures' can be transferred, to be stored until death. There are still some such hospitals functioning in the old ways but as Miss Doreen Norton points out in "*Hospitals of the Long-stay Patient*", their disintegration as functioning units is inevitable and, in some cases, imminent.

Nor, if one follows the story of Miss Phoenix through further, does it seem needful that there ever should have been these human warehouses. Roughly, the next stage is the advent of more activity into Miss Phoenix's annexe when occupational therapy was arranged twice a week. Miss Phoenix found that she had creative talent that she had not known about and she began to make things. This caused a great easing in our relationship. Now we had something other than pills to discuss when we met and it even proved possible to reduce the vast number she was on already. Miss Phoenix began to be a very different person, and I marvelled to see the change the OTs had wrought in someone with a degenerative condition such as hers. That summer the weather was good and it was possible to push Miss Phoenix into the garden, bed and all, and it seemed as though she was fulfilling one of our aims for our patients—namely that of living as fully as her disabilities permitted. Her family never honoured their promise to take her for drives and I did not press. I did not feel she was up to sitting in a car with comfort.

Then came a change in management. A new matron with different ideas and a supporting husband and family. She had been used to taking her patients out to see the Blackpool lights in her previous job. I riposted that Southend was fairly near, if she felt keen, and smiled at her jest. She challenged me, however, for permission to take them out if she could raise the money for a coach. I agreed, working on the policy that it is always better to say yes to a new idea, as one can get fused in one's thinking if one jolts along in a rut for too long. I thought also that she would be lucky if she managed to get many of the patients out in a coach, for a number of them had not even ventured into the garden for a long time, as they were extremely disabled.

It happened, however. The chaos of coffee mornings, handicrafts and sales and, *hey presto,* money for the coach. The quick check that medical permission was still forthcoming and a coach load of patients, relatives and staff were off to Whipsnade for the day—75 per cent of the patients. As the news broke that there was going to be a coach outing, Miss Phoenix wanted to know when and where and could she go? It was explained that the outing would entail sitting in the coach for six and a half hours and as she had not even sat in a chair for a few minutes for years, it was not possible for her to go. This roused her. She demanded to be sat out and gradually, in easy stages, was managing to be up for three hours by the day of the outing. Not enough. She was devastated, but by now she had the bit between her teeth and there was a purpose in life again. She started to get dressed; her hair was permed; she sat out in her chair all day; she tried a wheel-chair and liked it. We got her a self-propelling wheel-chair and despite her deformities and wasting, she began to move herself about the ward.

About this time, too, I had been listening to an officer of the

Wheel-Chair Section of the Ministry of Health saying that doctors rarely thought in terms of electric chairs for patients in the older age groups. Too true, one rarely did, as they are known to be very expensive pieces of equipment, but Miss Phoenix seemed to be a likely candidate. We put in a request and a few months later it came. She was thrilled beyond measure, even if it was a very fierce mechanism. By then she had been to a niece's wedding and done a trip to *The Black and White Minstrel Show* and had been up to London to see the Christmas lights. Life was looking up and she was on peak form.

For me there had had to be a good deal of re-thinking on this subject of the fallacy of inevitable deterioration. Dr. Binks had been putting forward this hypothesis for some time but it had not done more than rest delicately on the outer coverings of my intellect—seeing this miracle of fact unfolding before my eyes drove it through the layers with the force of a sledgehammer. Until then I had been concentrating my efforts (as far as my responsibilities lay with four long-stay annexes) in trying to bring life into the hospitals from the outside world and to relieve the tedium of existence by a steady inflow of different faces and things. This, I thought, would not only act as a tonic to the patients but would also in time relieve some of the load from the nurses.

Complacency was punctured yet again and another layer of habitual thought peeled off. Up to that point I had been a willing party to relatives taking patients home for the day or week-end, but there had always been a slight reservation when it came to longer periods. I knew it was illogical but it always seemed to me that if they could manage for a day or two, why not for good? Now I began to be much happier about a free-flow, with people deciding more for themselves when and how they could manage. Providing it did not disrupt the nurses' routine and make life more difficult for them, the more movement the better.

There is the mundane matter, of course, that if a hospital bed is empty, questions are always being asked as to why. I think it is this administrative and economic sword of Damocles hanging over many doctors' heads that makes them chary of permitting their patients much leave. In the same way, administrators of statutory social services are hamstrung by economics. One would expect that as their employers, the ratepayers, are also the consumers of the services provided, there would be a much closer correlation between need and provision. If Mrs. Feather and Miss Phoenix, particularly Mrs. Feather could have obtained the community help they required without delay, at the time they needed it, there is a likelihood that they need never have become long-stay hospital residents.

Unfortunately, Mrs. Feather, Miss Phoenix and their like do not constitute powerful or vocal forces in the voting community. Their plight tends to go unrecognised, concealed as it is beneath the smothering blanket of custodial care that is used to provide a solution for all individual problems of living. Their needs conflict economically with the pattern of the social services local authorities provide. Education, civic centres, playgrounds and similar matters are of more pressing import.

Too slowly is awareness coming that there is a crying need to co-ordinate and dovetail all social services in order to make them effective instruments of support for the individual, whether handicapped or old or both.

"The oldest hath borne most; we that
are young shall never see so much".
William Shakespeare

Reference

1. *The Care of Infirm Old People.* Report of a Study Group of the Standing Conference for Old People's Welfare (Gt. London) 1966. *Para.* 34.

Chapter Ten

PERSONAL CHOICE

"An intractable problem in the social services is the person who is always making demands but can never be satisfied with whatever is given".[1]

Said quickly, acceptance of people as they are is easy. For a doctor only seeing a patient infrequently, it is easier still. It is not so for nursing staff, coping day and night. And can we imagine what it is like to be almost buried alive? One meets and hears of 'difficult' patients, who are always being moved so that the strain of their support is distributed. They are usually labelled as "demanding", "interfering", "trying to run the ward" and so on. One such lady who is alert and intelligent is a great reader—despite complete paralysis. The only voluntary movement remaining allows her to flip over the pages of a book with one forefinger; this enables her to read, if the book-rest is adjusted precisely for her. Ten years of her life have been in a hospital ward and bed. Inevitably, she knows more of the ward routine than the constantly changing staff—being human she cannot forbear to advise occasionally! Inevitably, exasperation and frustration with her own predicament sometimes overflow and she is irritable. Unlike her attendants, she, who is at the mercy of those around her (even to having her nose wiped) cannot walk away from the situation; is it surprising she can be difficult? It is no surprise that now she is in an accepting place where her outbursts are understood they are fewer. Her family takes her out whenever they can, and the nurses go to endless trouble with her grooming; she appears to be in a state of equilibrium with her environment. Recollecting Miss Phoenix, who knows? One day some unexpected element may unlock resources previously unknown in her, and open up new vistas of living.

Such is one 'difficult' lady. Her history is ill recorded and I have no enthusiasm to upset the precarious balance in order to satisfy my curiosity.

MRS. NORTH's history is fuller and makes interesting reading. It leaves one feeling that a happier solution might have been reached, with more discussion and involvement all along the line.

Mrs. North was the twelfth child and pampered. Her much older husband continued the process. A friend supported her widowhood, lived with her, and helped run a small business. She died. Mrs. North kept on the house, but came south to spend long holidays with a younger relative. The age gap was minimal and both relative and husband were near retirement. A stroke, leaving a right hemiplegia, occurred on holiday. Some power returned to the leg and with the aid of a leg iron and tripod stick, she became *almost* independent. At this point her general medical ward 'hosts' became fearful lest she over-stay her welcome, and the medical social worker was detailed to arrange disposal. Coincidentally the husband had a stroke shortly after Mrs. North, and his wife could not manage two patients single-handed. Mrs. North wished to return to her north-country home, but the doctor pronounced that she must never again live alone. *Impasse.*

The medical social worker and relative decided on a private nursing home and the patient was transferred there acquiescently, whilst the relative went off to sell Mrs. North's house. The proceeds to be earmarked for the nursing home fees. During the month she was away, Mrs. North was totally without visitors. Soon after arrival, she had fallen trying to reach her commode unaided. Her customary apprehensiveness heightened and her morale reached zero. She was trapped in a situation far from her liking. The nursing home was not a good one. There was no alternative but to grit her teeth and await her relatives' return.

The pronouncement that an elderly person "must no longer live alone" is frequently made by doctors. Cataclysmic statement made, with equal frequency without regard to the long-term consequences, the doctor metaphorically washes his hands of the whole affair and family and friends are left to cope as best they may.

Selling up and moving to live with an offspring, *wherever* the latter may be, seem the only solution from an economic or accommodation view point. On our files, or occupying our long-stay beds, are many people whose ultimate breakdown in personal independence relates directly to uprooting from their native heath, hearth, contacts and environment. The moves were always planned with maximum good intent and sense of duty, but as the years passed total dependence and corrosion of relationships have occurred.

This is not surprising. It requires a very outgoing and mobile person to put down new roots and create the whole circle of things and people of which meaningful and satisfactory life is composed. Normally fresh contacts are made through the aid of definite work or social commitment. We find, however, that for such displaced and dispossessed elderly people—such as Mrs. North—the only human contacts tend to be the family and *their* friends. This sudden contraction of stimuli often culminates in withdrawal of the older person to room, then bed; with a concomitant increase of demands on the family. This in time becomes a vicious spiral. With less and less human contact and without the stimulation of variety in social exchange, the intellect begins to rust, and the mind to cloud over.

Reaching this stage the belated thought comes that life, with all its inherent dangers, would have been preferable in known familiar surroundings. After all, living itself is dangerous. Dying with one's boots on has greater dignity than rotting away slowly, cocooned in tender care, a passive object of familial solicitude and a source of increasing household tension.

The essence lies in Professor John MacMurray's words in *"Persons in Relation"* (1961) "My care for you is only moral if it includes the intention to preserve your freedom as an agent, which is your independence of me. Even if you wish to be dependent on me, it is my business for your sake to prevent it".

Mrs. North was moved to a nursing home run by a religious order. There, paradoxically, she had too much care. She had a room on her own, could stay in bed when she wished, and the bed-pan was brought if she did not feel like using the commode. She had no company and soon became depressed. She is typical of her stock—a shrewd, humorous, quick-fire repartee northerner with little intellectual resource and a great need for people.

Endeavours were made to get her into a Welfare Home nearer to her relatives. A new one opened close by and Mrs. North was one of the first residents. Her condition had already deteriorated, she had a urinary infection and, fearing to wet the bed, her need for bed-pans at night was so frequent, that after four months we were asked for help.

There was an embargo on admissions at that time for all but acute emergencies, and the referring practitioner was warned that a visit would not be followed by admission. Advice only would be possible, apart from out-patient help. He did not care; he was desperate. The Home staff were demanding action and his last effort had not had the desired effect. He had sent Mrs. North for investigation to a "genito-urinary chappie" he knew who was "awfully good" to his patients. Mrs. North had been admitted for three days only, examined, "no cancer found", bladder washouts recommended, but not done, and had been sent home precipitately. Several courses of antibiotics had been given without effect.

When the visit took place, the matron warned the visiting hospital physician that the situation could not be allowed to continue. Mrs. North was calling out for bed-pans twenty-five to thirty times a night and disturbing the other three patients in her room—altogether she was making a thorough nuisance of herself. She had not been incontinent. She was being wheeled everywhere in a wheel-chair of the type which is difficult for a disabled person to get in and out of without help and she was reputed to have done nothing for herself for weeks.

She was a very, very depressed woman and there are few more dismal sights than a bluff Northerner with the stuffing knocked out of her. She was apprehensive, morose and "can't" was her answer to most requests to demonstrate what she could do. She *could* actually walk quite well with a tripod but her shoes and iron and T-strap all needed a good deal of renovation.

The thing that struck the doctor most forcibly was the complete breakdown in relationships between patient and staff. The bell cord above her bed had been tied out of reach, to prevent her summoning the night nurses so often, and inevitably, she disturbed the other occupants of the room to get them to ring for her. There was a commode by her bed, which was 16 inches high, but her bed, at 22 inches, was too high for her to get in and out of to the commode without help. As the beds in the Home were of uniform height, nothing could be done about this. There was also a loose mat on the floor which was an added hazard.

We felt that immediate help was needed but there was no question of admission to hospital and even this would not alter Mrs. North's need for acceptance on her own terms and more encouraging management. We had few courses open to us. Firstly, we brought her up to the FAC to get to know her as a person on more neutral ground. Even this simple manoeuvre almost failed when the transport ordered did not arrive. Great pandemonium ensued on the telephone from the Home and the hospital doctor went to fetch her. Two of the Home's attendants saw her off, saying loudly to the doctor and within Mrs. North's hearing, "You can keep her. We do not want her back". She came again several times more but we always fetched her.

On other days we sent some of our therapy staff to the Home, hoping that by trying to restore Mrs. North's confidence in her own capabilities and in the full view of the Home's staff, some reconciliation might occur. This too was a dismal failure, particularly as Mrs. North managed to subside gracefully to the ground, just as the matron was passing! Worse still, Mrs. North had an incident of urinary incontinence during the daytime. There was no point in prolonging the struggle and by then the hospital staffing crisis had abated slightly and admitting could begin again.

Mrs. North came into hospital and a slow process of unthawing began. It took three weeks before she smiled—her only utterances consisted of incessant demands and the hospital night staff, like the night staff of the Home, led a miserable life. There is also the fact that we do not have an adequate number of adjustable height beds to give every person a bed at the right height for his need. Lavatories there are three—three for thirty patients. This whole medical block, opened just before the 1939-45 War, was designed for bedfast patients. At that time even three lavatories were considered to be almost gilt on the gingerbread. Commodes are few. Here again money to purchase an adequate number is a factor. Even if money could be raised—and this is feasible—there is not enough space in the wards to accommodate any more furniture and still leave enough working space for bedmaking and all the hundred and one activities that go on in a hospital ward. The ward is not only, in effect, a clinical working space where people receive technical, medical and nursing treatment but is also a place where people have to live.

Consequently, one is constantly being faced with the absurd dilemma, as with Mrs. North, that one brings patients into hospital in order to re-able them to independent living and yet the very physical properties and facilities available militate against this being achieved in any time shorter than a month of Sundays! (At least we have no problems with regard to tying up bell cords—there are no bells.)

As far as Mrs. North is concerned, at the time of going to press, she is a different person in many respects; lively—in fact too lively, for her tongue is never still. She is independent for most of her personal needs and by day she stomps out to the lavatory at will but at night we do not seem to have solved her difficulties. She is now more often than not incontinent, for she has great urgency and if she cannot get help at once it is usually too late. She has now come to accept this with an air of bravado—rather like an *enfant terrible*—which is her method of compensating for this awful piece of personal degradation in which, in spite of all her efforts, she has been forced to acquiesce. Furthermore, despite the fact that she now has more capital than she has ever had in her life, what good can it do her? She needs that which money cannot buy—the need to belong, to create, to give and to be needed. A place in the most opulent nursing home available will not help there. Our hospital may be poor in sheer civilised living conditions, but at least in it there is more possibility of fulfilling personal intangible needs than in many other institutional places.

Do our facilities need to be so limited? This opens up another era in the life of a physician working in the geriatric field. Until my ultimate end, I doubt whether I shall ever forget my first ward round in my first house physician's job in the professorial medical ward of my teaching hospital. Sister and I were making a quiet, preliminary round in the early morning, before the 'grand round' later with the whole flotilla of professor, staff and students. I innocently asked a man if he had had his bowels open as I knew the matter had been giving him much discomfort. Sister stopped her forward progress and with a marked politeness, asked me to leave the ward and come into her sitting-room. (No mere office at that time but the ward sister's centre of being—social and professional). I was touched that we should be having a coffee break so soon and followed her gaily into her room. As the door closed the storm burst—she was a first-class sister, a master of her craft, and was a great factor in training many green house physicians. She had also a good deal of Celtic blood. She was scarlet with rage and said cuttingly, "Doctor, please will you kindly attend to your medical concerns and I will attend to my nursing concerns". There followed an impassioned harangue, after which she swept out of her room to continue the round with apparent serenity, where we had left off. I hardly knew what had hit me but it made a great impression and from bowels and lavatories and all subjects pertaining to these mysteries in nursing, I kept my distance—until I came into geriatric work.

Someone has defined a geriatrician as being a catalyst of endeavour; others paraphrase Isaac Walton and think of him as the Compleat Physician, but it is a fact that in order to ensure that his patients have at least a reasonable slice of the cake, he has to be or become many things other than a doctor. He will start off in a small way when he puts in a requisition for a commode or new armchair for his ward. Back comes a memo, "What kind?" This is not just a delaying administrative tactic— and perforce there are many of these, for administrators lead an equally embattled life—but it is important that equipment should be correlated to needs. Miss Doreen Norton, in "*Hospitals of the Long-Stay Patient*", *Chapter VII*, 3.2, comments that there is a need for the application of ergonomics, which she defines as, having equipment which is designed for the task in hand, keeping in mind the capabilities of the person performing the task. An application as much needed by handicapped and aged infirm patients as by those who tend them.

Then, too, the geriatrician must become an expert in "committee poker". The old idea dies hard that geriatrics is a branch of medicine where nothing is being done for patients but the provision of custodial care and therefore very little expense should be incurred in the way of equipment, alterations or decor, and certainly there should be the minimum outlay on staffing. On the whole, the lay members of hospital committees are much in sympathy, albeit on a slightly sentimental basis, with the needs of geriatric departments. But it is not easy for them to balance the problem of priorities when it is a question, perhaps, of choosing between a kidney machine to save a life or new lavatories to help make the lives saved a bit more worth living. Administrators, too, have their problems, and it is not easy to withstand the demands and pressures from the more vocal and vigorous elements of the population and medical profession when questions of childbirth, coronary thrombosis, traumatic surgery, etc., are concerned. Seventy per cent of all adult admissions to district hospitals may be of the pensionable age group but it is not a vocal or adequately demanding group. Therefore, unless the administrator is having a specially far-seeing eye to the future, or else the physicians in charge of the geriatric departments can make their needs clearly and emphatically known and are willing to fight on every committee level for them, geriatric departments inevitably get only the crumbs from the rich, technical brother's table. Indeed, too excessive demands are being made on too limited resources.

Architecture featured nowhere in my medical education, but in recent years I have found myself having to spend more time making and studying plans than I have been able to spend reading my professional journals. Unless the syllabus has changed, there is also no time in a medical student's curriculum when he is instructed in the gentle art of writing long reports of the functions, limitations and future needs of his speciality. These are all matters which one thinks of happily as administration and not as part of a doctor's life. In this day and age of bureaucracy, however, this is not so. Unless one has the ability to describe in written detail and subsequently justify and defend in open committee the needs of one's department, one may just as well cease striving and either change one's occupation or else be content with the role that will be inevitably assigned to one—namely, that of being a clinical and administrative 'undertaker'.

An ordinary thinking member of the general public could be excused for being perplexed by this enigma. Here is this nationally known accepted fact, that we are an ageing population—one in five of us will be over pensionable age, and at risk—yet there is no clear lead or firm direction being given on the matter. The Ministry of Health suggests, the Regional Boards recommend, the Hospital Management Committees direct, those who are closest to the patients have to act as best they can, and the patient has to acquiesce in that which is offered and is available—choice is minimal.

The alternative is to have a wave of peristaltic action going the other way. Loud plaints and demands from patients' relatives to their elected representatives—insisting on more planning, better conditions, more staff and more scope for imaginative ways of dealing with people in need. The Ministry of Health should be leading and identifying needs, searching out how they are being best met and ensuring that the standards are brought up to those of the best, not levelled down. There is a need for clearing the brushwood and pruning back the administrative undergrowth that is beginning to strangle the Service.

With the proliferation of administrators and legislators in the last few decades, there appears to have been a great slowing up of the whole machine. Individuals are becoming afraid to act on their own responsibility. Initiation of new schemes is left to voluntary bodies to try out. Consequently, people with the more adventurous and creative talents go to work for the voluntary bodies and the schemes they produce tend to be discovered and used by like-minded clients. Inevitably, the statutory bodies and their more orthodox-minded employees are left to cope with the tougher problems of the non-spontaneous and inert. There is nothing to stop statutory bodies, except themselves and their own timidity, from being the innovators and initiators and from climbing out of the stultifying atmosphere of regulations.

One might postulate, of course, that patients receive the treatment they merit. One could take a small example of that very intimate thing—personal warmth. Some ten years ago, whilst working in another hospital group, one of my patients, who had been in hospital many years, a very disabled "burnt-out rheumatoid arthritic, who was an ex-JP and retained a very lively intellect and intact personality, suddenly developed a craving for a hotwater bottle. The ward had central heating but it was one of the old hutted emergency hospital buildings from the 1914-18 War and doubtless many sudden draughts assailed her at night. It may also have been that she was developing a widespread cancer that had not at that time shown itself clinically or it may have been that her only son was on parole after a long prison sentence and his frequent demands for money were making her small world feel very vulnerable. Whatever the cause, her need was clear and loudly expressed and I took up the campaign on her behalf. This is strictly a nursing concern in most hospitals, as any subsequent litigation following burns and scalds reflect on the nursing standards and therefore responsibility tends to rest on the chief nursing officer, not the medical staff. I took my plea to the chief nursing officer, and after some parleying an amicable agreement was made, for the patient to have her own thermostatically controlled electric blanket, of the type that goes over and not under the patient.

More recently, I had been involved with a fabulous 92-year-old, nearly blind lady, living at home in indescribable squalor although her means are far beyond those of the average person. She is an inveterate gambler and she still thinks nothing of winning £2,000 in a session at a gaming house. She is a lady who is very well-known to a number of hospitals and social services in the southern part of England, for she is, she says, campaigning for the rights of senior citizens. Her yardstick for testing the humanity of the hospitals she has cause to use from time to time is whether they will provide her with (*a*) privacy, and (*b*) a hot water bottle. In the last three years she has been referred to us twice. Each time she has been seen at home and each time she has clearly been in great need of hospital support; on each occasion we have been more than willing to offer it but on each occasion she has made her two requests, both on the face of it reasonable. The first time she was busy writing her memoirs and needed a single room in order that the marshalling of the affairs connected with this book should be possible and, at the same time, not too disturbing to other people in the ward. We had no such facilities to offer and she declined to come into this hospital.

On the more recent occasion she waived the room but was adamant on the hot water bottle to ease her aches and pains. Drugs had not the same effect, as she knew from experience, and in any case, they tended to have other unwished for side effects on her. No, a hot water bottle was her panacea. She knew the hospital regulations and questions of liability but she was willing to sign an undertaking accepting full responsibility for any eventualities. Once more, I took the problem to the chief nursing officer but with the passing of the years and further legislation, the official position had hardened. This rule was now inviolable and no exception could be made under any circumstances. So once more the effect of a few patients or relatives suing over results of accidents which had happened when action had only been taken with good intent had meant preclusion of personal comfort for many others. Perhaps if relatives or patients sued because of lack of adequate lavatory accommodation or washing facilities or the dearth of beds of the right height, this might produce positive rather than negative legislation. It would give fresh heart to and embolden the people actually administering such legislation, to vary the rules to fit the person. So often nowadays we seem to be following the methods of Procrustes, the innkeeper of the Greek fable, who, by the process of stretching or lopping off the legs of shelter-seeking travellers, made them fit the inn's one bed.

"There's place and means for every man alone".
William Shakespeare

Reference

1. *The Care of Infirm Old People.* Report of a Study Group of the Standing Conference for Old People's Welfare (Gt. London) 1966. *Para.* 22.

Chapter Eleven

IMPERATIVE RELEGATION

> *"This describes a method of approach which assumes that certain people must be consigned to a somewhat less important sphere. It also assumes that the person consigned will naturally accept this and those to whom the person is consigned will naturally be there to accept, without question, total responsibility".*[1]

This is a subject we have touched on several times already—namely, the way specialist and teaching hospitals, situated at a distance from where people live, irresponsibly and unthinkingly relegate certain patients to the geriatric hospital nearest to the patient's home. These are the patients for whom it is deemed "no more can be done".

It seems inevitable, in the high order of scientific specialisation that has developed in the second half of this century, that there are bound to be certain centres of specialisation. Not every district hospital can support the provision of neuro-surgical, organ replacement, plastic surgery, radiotherapy departments or the like. Inevitably there will have to be regional centres for such, but it does seem imperative that except in cases of emergency, it would be best if referrals to such centres were made from the district hospital. It would then, perhaps, prevent the heartburnings such as have occurred in some of the cases previously outlined, as there would be a clear responsibility chain. There is also need to hasten the trend for ensuring that teaching hospitals take district hospital responsibility for the area in which they are situated. Then instead of concentrating the numbers of highly trained staff in their own specialised precincts, these could be shared with the present district hospitals where there is an even greater need. One recollects hearing of the famous old teaching hospital being asked to write a treatise on the rehabilitation of stroke patients. This produced a degree of embarrassment to the extremely competent people concerned, for rarely did they have more than two stroke patients in the whole hospital or out-patient departments at a time. Their hospital did not have district responsibility and the admissions were therefore of a highly selective nature, and unless the patient more or less had a stroke on the premises such an ordinary run of the mill condition was never likely to find its way into the wards. This hospital had a complement of up to thirty physiotherapists.

Let us then consider the case of *MRS. SMILER* who was attending a teaching hospital where there is a complement of sixty trained physiotherapists and an attached School of Physiotherapy.

Mrs. Smiler had been referred to the teaching hospital ten years before we knew about her troubles and for ten years she had been attending there as an in-patient and out-patient, having various surgical procedures done and being an excellent case for demonstration, teaching and examination purposes. She had tremendous faith and trust in the hospital which gave her most competent and kindly care at all levels. After ten years of this happy relationship, it suddenly struck her medical advisers that Mrs. Smiler was fast becoming a long-term hospital problem and if they were not careful they were going to have her 'blocking' one of their beds. The registrar of the firm concerned was therefore detailed off to obtain her admission to a chronic-sick unit in her home area. He wrote a long letter listing all the technicalities of her condition and ended up with an ambiguous statement to the effect that she was looked after in her own home by her aged husband and the district nurse.

Our administrative doctor wrote back to enquire more as to the actual function of the patient and the plans and actions that must have undoubtedly been initiated to make management at home as realistic as possible. If they had now reached a point where they considered Mrs. Smiler needed a hospital environment and they expected the decision to be implemented by others, then we would need to see the patient and assess the situation ourselves, in which case we would need to have a request from the family doctor.

At this point came a report from the medical social worker to explain the original medical request. The medical social worker explained Mrs. Smiler's mental and physical deterioration, her immense weight and her need for five people to lift her as she could not be managed with a hoist. She was receiving intensive passive and active physiotherapy, and although she had a wheel-chair, she could rarely be put into it. Occupational therapy was not possible for her because she had no control over her hands and she lacked mental concentration. It was further apparent that she was still in the teaching hospital.

Later, the registrar reported progress. Mrs. Smiler had lost weight and could now stand and take a few steps with the help of three physiotherapists.

We responded that if this was the case, Mrs. Smiler was, according to her needs, in the right place. We had one part-time physiotherapist and it was unlikely that five people would ever be available to lift her.

It was possible to visit Mrs. Smiler when she was moved to the hospital's convalescent annexe nearer to our area and fortuitously her husband was visiting at the same time. Much polite discussion occurred and it seemed as though there was a possibility at last of arranging to act in concert with the teaching hospital—they using their technical resources of time and personnel and we using our local knowledge of domestic resources. Accordingly, we wrote to suggest this symbiotic approach—in short, that they should make Mrs. Smiler wheel-chair independent and abandon the walking attempts that were clearly never going to pay dividends. Meanwhile, we would visit the house and, keeping in touch with their ancillary staff, make sure that the patient's needs in the way of hoists, ramps and other modifications were ready to receive her on her return home. We would then take over her support on an out-patient basis. We had tentatively discussed this plan with both patient and husband and the convalescent annexe staff when assessing the patient, and all had viewed it with favour. Not so our medical colleagues who came to the conclusion that we must have seen her on her "best day for months." Naturally they were aiming at wheel-chair independence but they could not see this stage being possible for four to five years at the earliest, and sending her home to her frail old husband would result in disaster to him.

We wondered whether the fact that it was her "best day for months" might have been produced by Mrs. Smiler seeing a slight hope of returning home, but we now realised that symbiotic action was unlikely. We accepted that inevitably, if Mrs. Smiler were to be returned home, we would have to be the agents to implement it and it would have to be when the time was optimum from our point of view, for Mrs. Smiler's own sake. We had no illusions about the time and energy that would have to go into this undertaking. We were also well aware, from similar undertakings in the past, what misery patients experience from feelings of rejection and the contrast in material amenities when coming from a teaching to a less well-endowed hospital.

Soon came a peremptory letter from the world-famous physician under whose care she was, demanding removal of Mrs. Smiler from his bed, which she had occupied for too long, to one of our long-stay beds. Shades of Poor Law once more! It is hard for one brought up in the days of this Act to appreciate fully that 1948 and the National Health Service inauguration changed all the imperative legislation. It was obvious from the tone of his letter that Mrs. Smiler could expect nothing more than custodial care in her present situation and if there were ever to be any possibility of return home, we would have to act as the agents, and fast.

As Dr. Binks has frequently mentioned, it is strange that though no one would expect any but the surgeon in charge to decide whether or not an operation is to be performed, a sense of incongruity never strikes those who solemnly pronounce that long-stay hospital accommodation must now be given but who are not prepared to give it. In other words, they are perfectly prepared to commit someone else to a course of action they are unwilling themselves to pursue. Was it Johnson who described power without responsibility as being the prerogative of the harlot down the ages?

There seems little to be gained by going into a long description of how Mrs. Smiler was re-abled to return home. It took six months of hard slog on the part of everyone concerned, the work being made much harder by the fact that Mrs. Smiler was unaware of the true diagnosis of her complaint. Also, that she had been conditioned by the intensive passive and active physiotherapy to the belief that if she were given enough of this, and often enough, she would be able to walk again and then there would be no problem. She was, therefore, resentful of the fact that batches of physiotherapists did not appear as heretofore, to put into operation the elaborate ritual of her 'walking' exercise.

Though mechanical problems—the right wheel-chair, adaptations to the house, arrangements with the welfare authorities, obtaining more help in the house, working out dressing problems, activities, and how to turn her in bed and get her to a sitting position in bed—took endless time, the main stumbling block to the whole operation 'Return Home' was bowel regulation.

Here it might be appropriate to comment on this subject. One of my social worker colleagues once described geriatric work as "life lived at lavatory level"—what a true aphorism. We always point out to students that in biblical times the bowels were described as the seat of emotions. It was the Victorians who started the cult of the heart being the organ of emotion. Perhaps this is true of the superimposed emotions but there is no doubt that for a sense of true well being the regulation of bowel function is intrinsic!

Physiologically, there seems to be a strange unawareness in some elderly people (though this is not unknown in busy and otherwise occupied younger ones) that the bowel is gradually silting up. They may have a small amount of action infrequently and consider it to be adequate and commensurate with their current dietary intake. Then they may have some episodes of faecal incontinence which they are unable to control. This may at first be attributed to an attack of diarrhoea and may pass. There may be concomitant episodes of abdominal pain and vomiting or transient confusion, and the whole cycle of events may be repeated numerous times before help is sought.

The causes leading to such constipation are various. We also consider it to be an occupational hazard of any resident in any form of institution, i.e. hospital, Home or hostel or hotel or even hall of residence, where food and fluid intake is not regulated by personal choice and predilection but dictated by the overall catering service of the institution. In an ordinary home one can obtain a drink without thought and there is usually ready access to water. In institutional life this is more difficult. For a non-ambulant patient the intake of fluid is first limited by availability and the ability to take it unaided but also voluntary limitations are frequently effected, particularly by women, in an endeavour to cut down the need for bed-pans or trips to the lavatory. Lack of fluid, immobility and limited roughage are well-known precursors of constipation: less well known, perhaps, are the effects of many drugs. Codeine compounds are consumed in quantity, but how many people think of its binding properties? Fortunately, the current popular panacea, paracetamol, has more tendency to produce loose stools. Most of the popular drugs for night sedation are also costive in action.

The physiological phenomenon of the pseudo-diarrhoea produced by impacted faeces is again not often included in medical or nursing curriculi, and yet, it is one of the most important features of hospital life at all ages from the point of view of patient comfort and general well-being. Very simply, the rectum becomes blocked by a hard mass or masses of faecal matter and this mass will distend the rectum and stretch the anal sphincter so that it is incapable of contracting tightly as it normally does, to hold back even a fluid stool. Higher up the pelvic colon, the intestinal contents (more fluid normally), dammed back will liquefy further through the action of the bacteria. The liquid stool then seeps down round the mass blocking the rectum and seeps out uncontrollably through the anus, producing the apparent diarrhoea. Too often this will be treated as true diarrhoea and quantities of gumming-up potions will be consumed which will aggravate the whole situation. Like poor Mrs. Milliner (*Chapter Four*), such cases are at risk of being whisked into hospital as acute abdominal emergencies.

One thinks wistfully that if one had been paid in guineas for all the bizarre conditions which one has been instrumental in 'curing' by merely relieving constipation, one would long since have been able to retire in peace to a sunny clime where the wine, the fruit and the oil used in the cooking preclude this strange ailment of the cold carbohydrate-loving countries of the northern hemisphere.

This may not be a 'nice' subject and its discussion may be considered out of place except in medical and nursing manuals, but why should this be so? This is a subject that very intimately concerns us all; furthermore, it is an ailment whose remedy lies in our own hands, be we but aware of it. And how are we to be aware of it but by free discussion? Even doctors who are considered by their peers to excel in the field of care of old people have been known to be oblivious to the simple facts of life with regard to pseudo-diarrhoea. Take one general practitioner of my acquaintance who is the visiting physician to a number of Old People's Homes in this area. He is considered to be such an expert in his work that he was sponsored on a trip abroad to study Old People's Homes there. Yet he referred a resident of one of the Homes to our out-patient clinic "query carcinoma of the colon with secondaries". The symptoms? "Intractable faecal incontinence over several months and now presenting with a mass in her abdomen. In the past she has been in a mental hospital and is senile".

A thin old lady with an unhappy facial tic and a somewhat difficult speech impairment appeared in the clinic. She was alone and therefore time had to be spent on establishing communication and learning about her. Gradually the story unfolded; of rejection by her husband, causing her admission to an Old People's Home after her discharge from the mental hospital—sufferance there—little activity—lifelong constipation—confinement to bed with an acute infection, and gradual onset of unwonted 'dirtiness' which had upset her very much. She had never soiled herself or her bed at all before and she was ashamed and embarrassed. She was equally proud that despite this she was in complete control of her water and had never *wet* her bed.

The story spoke for itself. I was fairly sure what I would find when I came to examine her. And it was so. She was thin and her abdomen, on palpation, was a mass of hard lumps—indeed, if carcinoma it had been, it would have been of the galloping variety! On rectal examination there was a huge mass of rocklike faeces distending her rectum, rather reminiscent of a foetal skull. We will draw a veil over the battle to relieve that followed. It was too uncomfortable for patient and operator. Suffice is to say that 4½ lbs. of hard rocks were delivered. She might easily have had some other pathology but in that state it was impossible to tell. I telephoned the matron of the Home and was not surprised to hear that she had been put on a low roughage diet, kept off fluid and been dosed with vast quantities of Kaolin and morphine. She would need to reverse the treatment, and the patient was to return to the clinic in two weeks when the bowels were clear to be re-examined. A colleague saw her and removed 2½ lbs. more rocks which were blocking the rectum and noted that there were still rocks palpable in the abdomen. "Continue laxatives and return in two weeks' time" was the suggestion. I saw her again. By this time there were no masses to feel in her abdomen but rocks still had to be removed in the final clearance of the rectum, i.e. one month or four weeks after commencement of rigorous disimpaction treatment. This is an irrefutable example to quote to anyone who thinks to cure faecal impaction with one enema or washout or a couple of suppositories.

Reverting to Mrs. Smiler who had just such problems. Owing to her paralysis, she had little or no feeling of her bowel state and consequently would have no warning. Her husband, though willing to undertake any task, found that clearing up after these incidents was something he could not do as a routine: it sickened him too much. This seemed fair (I could well sympathise myself—I have never been able to cope with bed-pan emptying!) In a teaching hospital Mrs. Smiler's bowels had been dealt with once a week. On 'Bowels Day' she had been incommunicado—no visitors—no nothing. We could not quite understand this when she was transferred to us, but when the enormousness of her action became manifest on 'Bowels Day', we appreciated why she suffered so much and was then too exhausted to receive visitors. We felt that twice or thrice weekly actions would be less exhausting and more normal, and after some trial and error, twice weekly was found to suit her best. The question then was, as with Mrs. Wilholm (*Chapter Five*) how to make this happen at a predictable time, for, like Mrs. Wilholm, the problem of her passing urine was taken care of by a self-retaining catheter.

This was the problem on which everything hinged, for her maintenance at home was dependent upon her husband and he would manage, and manage well, with support coming in, as long as he did not have to cope with the problem of bowel actions. Therefore, her rhythm had to be tuned in with a visit from the district nurse or the very excellent home help. On this hung everything and on this we were hung up for weeks. Then, as with Mrs. Wilholm, we thought we had achieved a pretty fool proof rhythm by giving laxative granules the night before bowels day at a fixed time and the district nurse calling and giving a special type of suppository at 9 am. This happened on the ward fairly successfully and on the occasions when Mrs. Smiler went home on trial to make sure all was well. There was nothing left to do now but try it out, so when everyone concerned, from family doctor and district nurse to welfare officer for the physically handicapped, had thought all contingencies had been considered and provided against as far as humanly possible, she went home.

A copy of the discharge summary to the family doctor was sent as a matter of courtesy to the teaching hospital physician. He responded lightly by writing that he now knew the most effortless way of getting his problem cases re-established at home. By then we had a fair amount of 8 mm. cine film recording the means and methods used in this task and indicating some of the trials and tribulations involved. We wrote suggesting that a meeting of the teaching hospital team and the geriatric team, who had both been concerned with Mrs. Smiler's welfare, might be profitable in order to discuss Mrs. Smiler's case and their common problems and function. We felt that in view of all the previous correspondence, this would be the only way that the two sides would come to have any knowledge and respect for each other's work and facilities. The letter still remains unanswered.

"A rainbow and a cuckoo's song may never come together".
W. H. Davies

Reference

1. Binks, F. Allen. (1968). *Brit. Med. J.*, **i**, 269-74

Chapter Twelve

THE COMMUNITY

> *"We are often led to believe that most of our troubles are due to some dramatic social change, as the result of which families no longer look after their old people".*[1]

This is the easiest form of rationalisation there is, but there have been enough examples quoted already, one hopes, to refute this.

If one looks back into the early centuries when there were far fewer elderly people alive, one finds writers deploring the fact that families would not look after their old folk. Canon Barnett was complaining about his parishioners' heartlessness in the 19th century and in 17th century England "widowed mothers could not always rely on their children to give them a home."

What then are the main factors contributing to the present conditions? Where are the main inadequacies occurring in the Welfare State?

From our point of view there seem to be two very specific and important areas where there are glaring deficiencies:—

1) Housing.
2) Retirement according to age, without adequate preparation.

First let us consider housing. Two cases stand out in my mind—one successful and one unsuccessful—neither atypical.

The first was the minute *MR. JACKO,* 64 when he first came in as an emergency through the Casualty Department. He sold newspapers outside a tube station. He had no kith and kin. He was 4 feet 9 inches high and had huge dark eyes. His whole appearance, when he was well, was rather reminiscent of a friendly monkey. When he was ill his eyes were small black dabs on huge white saucers. He lived in digs (condemned property) and he was in and out of hospital frequently with exacerbations of his chronic bronchitis, mainly brought on by malnutrition and inadequate and cold housing. He frequently wintered in hospital, spinning out his symptoms until the warmer weather came. When his chest troubles cleared up, he would produce symptoms of a peptic ulcer and he would appear to be in such pain and agony that frequent resort was made to milk drips. After several such admissions, we tried to support him with daily attendances to the ward for group occupational activity and a midday meal, but even this was not successful, so the welfare authorities were asked to see him with a view to finding him other accommodation. They offered him a place in one of their Homes, which he accepted. At that time the Middlesex County Council had one Residential Home at the seaside in Norfolk. Mr. Jacko agreed to go, for he had no family ties and it sounded pleasant to go to the seaside. However, he was a Cockney sparrow and did not transplant, and soon he was back in London and back in hospital. After this he had a spell at Springbok House whilst fresh thought was being given to the problem of accommodation and he enjoyed this even more than hospital.

He then went into sheltered housing. The Borough Council had taken over several houses in a row and turned them into bed-sitting rooms with shared kitchen and bathroom facilities and a resident warden in attendance. Mr. Jacko throve better there and his hospital admissions were reduced.

Then there came a gap of two years when we did not see him. We concluded that he must have died or left the district, but he reappeared on the 8th December one year with a severe bout of broncho-pneumonia. We were not surprised as Mr. Jacko loved Christmas in hospital and his joy in the ward festivities was always recompense for the staff. On antibiotics, he picked up quickly, but to our intense surprise he began to agitate for his discharge. He simply had to get out before Christmas, he said. He had so many pre-Christmas engagements and he did not wish to miss anything. There was a trip to the pantomime—an outing there—a dinner here—a party elsewhere. So home he went. It was noted somewhat belatedly that his address was different from that of the last admission.

The next time he was seen was a coincidence. The Council had built a whole new block of one-roomed flats for elderly people, with a resident warden and communal sitting rooms. There were cooking and washing facilities in the rooms but shared bathrooms. The residents 'did' for themselves, but help was at hand if needed, by pressing a bell. Background central heating was included in the rent, but best of all, they could take their own furniture.

Whilst visiting a critically ill old man one bitter winter's day in one of these flatlets, I asked who did the shopping, etc., for him. He said that a friend down the corridor did it, and as an afterthought suggested that the friend might be known to me as he had been in our hospital many times. It was, of course, Mr. Jacko. I went along and knocked at his door which was ajar and the most happy sight imaginable met my eye when I pushed open the door. There was Mr. Jacko sitting in his armchair by his electric fire—these were supplied in all the rooms to boost the heating as needed. His thumbs were stuck in his waistcoat armholes and he was smoking a cigar almost as big as himself it seemed, with an expression of utter bliss and contentment on his face. He had found himself at last. He had his own home; he was warm; he had found his own niche, for he was depended upon and needed. I have often seen him since when visiting in the area, even on the coldest day, out shopping, doubtless for people more disabled than himself. He is now over 70 and getting a trifle portly but he has not needed hospital treatment again for over two years. If for some reason he does develop a further exacerbation of his bronchitis (too much smoking of cigars perhaps?), hospital admission, I warrant, would only be a brief incident in his busy life. As on the last occasion, he will not stay one moment longer than is needful.

If only there were more such flatlets, where people could take their own belongings and maintain their independence but with some support and the option of companionship; where that most vital element—background heating—is laid on automatically and not as an extra. These flatlets should not be tucked away from the road, uphill or a mile from the nearest shops, as is one new development in this area. Our forebears showed infinite wisdom in building small groups of almshouses on main streets where there is much activity and access to shops is simple. This type of dwelling, modernised, is still the most popular accommodation there is, and one can be fairly sure that any person from one of these who comes into hospital will not remain willingly for a day longer than is necessary. The LCC built a block of flatlets near a new residential Home in Hackney. This was part of an experiment, for it was expected that the infirm tenants from the flats would progress to the Home. Surprisingly, it was found that in the first six years none did so; furthermore, the matron at the Home, who also acted as warden for the flats, preferred to nurse any ill tenants in their own flats instead of in the sick bay of the Home, as had been planned. She said that they recovered much faster in their own surroundings.

The redoubtable *MRS. STALWART* was not so fortunate. She was 85 when she first came into hospital with gangrene of her toes and by the time she was transferred to a 'chronic surgical bed' and we came to nodding acquaintance with her she had been in hospital eighteen months and had lost both legs by stages. Despite her age she had insisted on new legs being provided, and was struggling to adapt herself to two full-length prostheses—a formidable task even for a younger person. Normally she lived alone in a small house packed with furniture. She had agreed to sell it and had opted for a council ground floor flat. Reluctantly, she let her family sell up and move her things for her; she hated not being able to see to things herself. In the meantime, she toiled away at making herself independent in a wheel-chair and trying to master the incorrigible legs, fuming all the while at the slowness of the housing authorities. She could not see why they had not provided enough flats or bungalows for handicapped people like herself. Surely, she reasoned, she was not unique.*

She was allocated a ground floor old people's flat. There was the inevitable step to the front door. A ramp could not be made

*Rankin & Weir 1967. Inquiry into the Incidence of Chronic Illness and Disability in the Young and Middle-aged.

"There are believed to be about 370,000 handicapped people of working age alone in Great Britain at the present time".

because it was one of a row in which all the front doors opened on to a narrow communal walk. Therefore she could not propel herself in and out of the front door in her wheel-chair. Nor was there much future as far as the french window at the back was concerned, for it opened on to the grass and she was unable to move her chair across the soft ground. Consequently, once in the flat she was a prisoner.

The lavatory was too low; the sink and kitchen surfaces were the wrong height for her wheel-chair, and in any case her chair would not go through the doorway into the kitchen. In order to pull herself up from her chair to her legs she needed a very stout handrail fixed to the wall. Owing to regulations which have been mentioned before, with regard to Mrs. Wilholm (*Chapter Six*) none of these alterations could be carried out until she was registered as physically handicapped. This could only be done at home. At that time she was not one of our patients and our acquaintance was only social. However, our staff and their friends were her best clients, for she spent her waking time making very gorgeous lamp shades.

Despite all her problems, she very determinedly went off to her new home, leaving her legs behind her in the Physiotherapy Department where she was reunited with them at regular intervals as an out-patient. As an out-patient she used to struggle along between the parallel bars, patiently awaiting the day when a bar would be installed for her in the flat and she could then take her legs home and be able to pull herself up on to them and walk about to do her chores.

With the help of her family, who did the shopping and housework and saw to her fires (no background heating here), she managed three months in the flat without her legs. No mean feat this when one considers that she had to get up on an average three times each night, transferring from bed to wheel-chair, to lavatory, back to wheel-chair and back to bed. Retrospectively, one wonders why no one thought of a commode chair by the bed. It was on one of those nightly trips that the brake of her wheel-chair slipped, precipitating Mrs. Stalwart on to the floor. She was not to be defeated without a fight and she tried, by piling up all available cushions and pillows, to form a sort of ladder to get herself back into bed again. She did not manage this and had to remain on the floor all night, awaiting help.

It was winter and, as her son was to remark rather bitterly at a later stage, the only adaptation that had been done to the flat was to remove the door between the bed-sitting room and the kitchen, which meant that there was always a howling gale sweeping through the room. She developed broncho-pneumonia; her spirit was temporarily broken and back she came into hospital, to a general medical ward. There, in her despondency, she submitted to persuasion and wearily agreed to make an application for admission to a designated Welfare Home. Meanwhile, the Geriatric Department had been asked to take her over, the referral note reading, "This lady has bilateral amputations and cannot be helped by her family. There is no medical treatment and the problem is to find institutional care for her".

We did take her over and by then, having recovered her spirit (despite painful pressure sores), Mrs. Stalwart was agitating once more for re-housing in accommodation properly adapted for her. She had written to her Borough Councillor on a number of occasions, asking him to come and see her to discuss her needs but had met with no response. We had meetings with the patient, family and welfare authorities but there was no other suitable housing known to be available in the whole borough. When Mrs. Stalwart saw there was no alternative, she agreed to compromise by looking at the accommodation being offered in a new residential Home. If she liked it, she agreed to go there temporarily as long as she would be allowed to continue her campaign of agitation to persuade the Borough Councillors to get proper accommodation planned and built for herself and people like her.

The matron of the Home came to see her and they liked each other. Mrs. Stalwart then went to see the Home and the matron, with great humanity and courage, offered to house her prized sideboard and some of her choicest ornaments in the Home (strictly against regulations) until such time as she found her own place. As there were some single rooms, it was possible for Mrs. Stalwart to have one and be independent at night with a commode by her bed. Still protesting about the unfairness of community arrangements, she went off but, despite her efforts, she got no response to her lobbyings, and her very great spirit broke. She hated the residential home life where there was no purposeful activity to occupy her days and she eventually gave up the struggle. She took to bed and after five months she was back with us, unconscious. A fortnight later she died.

She was right. She was far from being unique. There are many with needs precisely the same as hers and too little is being done to meet them.

MRS. KEEPER-JONES, was a widow, living on a pittance and National Assistance in a block of flats. So keen was she to remain at this good address that she lived without heat or light and almost without food in order to do so. When the rent went higher and the Assistance Board refused to meet the difference any longer and insisted on her applying for an Old People's Home, she gave up. Needless to say, it was to hospital she came and it was there she died a few months later.

Coincidentally, *MR. BACKER* was a neighbour of Mrs. Keeper-Jones in this same block of flats. His wife did dressmaking at home and they made ends meet financially. His problem was uncomplicatedly one of failure to prepare for retirement.

He had been an exceptionally fit man all his life. He had never been off sick from work and he had gone on working as a storekeeper with a car firm until he was 68. Normally the employees of this firm were automatically retired at 65 and they considered that they had been kind to allow him to go on until he was 68. The chopper came eventually, after an amalgamation. He was filled with resentment—the more so when he found his income sadly reduced. His only hobby apart from work had been going out with his friends to sporting events and pubs. As his finances now precluded him standing his rounds, despite his friends' assurances that it need make no difference, he ceased to go out with them : in fact, from the day of his retirement until going into hospital thirteen years later he never crossed the threshold out of his flat.

Very shortly after retirement he developed a pain in his chest, diagnosed by his too sympathetic doctor as a coronary thrombosis. He was put to bed and kept there for six months, with his wife waiting on him hand and foot. After this he developed sciatica and arthritis. He consumed so much aspirin to relieve his pains that he had a haematemesis and had to be admitted to hospital. The aspirin was stopped and he went on a codeine derivative. At home again, he found it difficult to move about and stopped in his bedroom all day and every day. When it became painful to lie in bed because of his hip, he lay half in and half out of bed, with one leg down on a footstool. He developed postural oedema and the skin of his leg ulcerated. Then one night he went to the kitchen to wash his teeth, as he usually did at 2 am, and lost his balance and fell. It took three neighbours to get him back to bed.

When the doctor saw him next day, he decided that it was heart failure and put him on massive doses of digoxin and very powerful diuretics. When he was seen two weeks later, he was in a very parlous state indeed, suffering from tremendous nausea, dizziness and ringing in his ears from the high digoxin doses. The powerful diuretics had dehydrated him and also made him unable to control his micturition and he had to sit with a urinal at the ready the whole time. He was still suffering from pain from the fall and he was admitted as quickly as possible to hospital, for a fractured femur seemed a likely possibility and he needed to have his drug treatment reduced drastically.

His response to a new environment was dramatic and his complete reversal from dejected misery to spontaneous brightness was a pleasure to behold. Unfortunately, or perhaps fortunately, for it is difficult to see how the clock could have been put back in Mr. Backer's case, or indeed how some more satisfying way of life could have been found for him when he went home again, he died suddenly in his sleep one night.

His case was a little unusual, perhaps, in that he never went out again following his retirement, but he managed to maintain an intact personality and he had some intellectual resources as he became a great reader and listened to sporting events on the radio.

The little man who walked into the clinic one morning and burst into tears was a different sort of personality. His doctor's letter of introduction said, starkly, "Senile dementia. Please see and advise". There was an anecdote when I was a student, of a doctor who used to send patients along to the hospital with no more introduction than the doctor's visiting card with "Please see" written on the back. On one occasion he received a reply on the same card, returned by the incensed hospital surgeon, with the simple inscription, "Have seen"! When I read the doctor's letter before the patient was shown in, I had been planning a reply on these lines but on seeing *MR. POLLY*, these fanciful thoughts went. He appeared, and was, an exceptionally fit and well preserved 68-year-old. He sobbed so much that I gave up trying to get his story from him and turned to the accompanying son. Poor Mr. Polly had been axed from his government job at 65. It was a simple manual labouring job but he had been a good workman. He had no friends or hobbies other than keeping pigs in his back garden. This gave him great satisfaction and was a good help to the household economy. It was a somewhat unusual urban hobby, one would imagine. This kept him going quite happily for the first two years of his retirement until the landlord sold half of the garden and it was no longer possible to keep the pigs. There was nothing left for Mr. Polly. He sat at home, got under his wife's feet, followed her about and eventually he sobbed whenever she left him alone. Her temper gave out and she summoned the doctor and told him that something must be done. It was. We were it.

There seemed no solution to this one. Physically he was very healthy, but as I sat gazing at his notes, hoping for inspiration, I noticed his address and remembered that he must live near to a Workroom for Elderly People which had opened not long before. He did, and the son knew it well but had never thought of his father going there. This all took place on a Saturday morning. The following Wednesday, when making my first visit to see this new Workroom, one of the first people I saw there was Mr. Polly, happily engaged on one of the simpler repetitive jobs. He did well; the discipline of regular work again, saved his tottering reason and his wife always placed herself outside the Workroom entrance to collect his pay packet from him when he came out on pay days.

There are so many people of Mr. Backer's and Mr. Polly's generation and type who need either the status and financial reward that goes only with work, or who need the simple discipline of having some objectives for which to get up and dress and shave and go out. For many, a work situation is the only thing that answers this need. We are a work orientated society.

The subject of retirement is one that is being opened up all too slowly. There is a Pre-Retirement Association in the United Kingdom but it has almost expired from lack of financial support. It should be getting moral and economic support of every kind, not only from industry but from the government and community at large. Money spent on encouraging preparation for retirement and providing sheltered work shops and work centres and adequate housing would drastically reduce the tremendous health and welfare sums now devoted to providing institutional custodial care. It would be difficult to bring definite statistical figures to support this contention as it is virtually impossible to relate prevention to cure. It is a statement that can only be made by retracing the histories of the majority of people who become long-stay patients in hospital or residents of old people's Homes.

"We know what we are but know not what we may be".
William Shakespeare

Reference

1. Binks, F. Allen. (1968). *Brit. Med. J.*, **i**, 269-74.

Chapter Thirteen

THE TEAM

"If we do the right thing for the right reason, other things have a tendency to fall into place: 'truth has always a certain clarity of line'".[1]

This causerie started out as a description of how one particular geriatric unit goes about its business. No two such units will ever tackle problems in precisely the same way because no two units ever have the same circumstances in which to operate. Given a different area and unified accommodation, we would probably function in some other manner, but it seems likely that there are certain elements that are essential in order to function at all in any set of circumstances.

The first and primary essential is to have a medical director of considerable clinical and intellectual calibre who has also sufficient integrity of purpose to be able to withstand the multiple and varied vested interests that assail him from his appointment day onwards. But however firm of resolve he may be, he will accomplish little until he has acquired about him a collection of people of varying disciplines but either of similar ways of thought, or, at least, with open and flexible enough minds to be willing to join the struggle to "find the clarity of line".

The descriptions through these pages have come as through the perception of one of the doctors of a team that has been collecting round the Physician-in-Charge of the Geriatric Unit at Edgware over the years. The expression is specific to one person; this is how things seem to me, but many of the thoughts expressed have evolved from the unending discussions that go on between all of us who work in the Unit which started as a fragmented dissociate conglomerate—a many-headed multitude—but which very slowly is beginning to find some sort of composite form. This is due to the fact that there is team-work, not in theory but in genuine hard fact. Team-work is a very fashionable word. Every industry, business concern, educational or government establishment stresses the need for team-work, but to produce real team-work calls for far more from the people concerned than is ever imagined.

Communication between human beings can never be easy; communication between people with widely differing training and mostly with developed and strong personalities requires much resilience, for very few gravitate to geriatrics when newly hatched from their professional training, nor is it often advisable. The stresses and strains involved require more mature experience.

If one is status seeking or status conscious, one can never fit into a team framework; one's ego would be pricked too incessantly to be able to withstand the strain. In a true team there is no status and no hierarchic structure; there are no lines of demarcation except on merit. To be a worthwhile instrument, the team must have true regard and respect for each other's worth and potential, and arising from their contact with each other, they must be prepared for interchange of role. Many occasions will arise when a doctor must be prepared to act or think in speech therapy terms, for instance; the medical social worker like a physiotherapist; the physiotherapist like a medical social worker; the occupational therapist think in medical terms, and so on. All must be prepared to put themselves in the place of the patient and his relative. If one is jealous of one's disciplinary training and status, then such interplay can never be accepted or tolerated. Fortunately, where the sole aim is to support people to regain independence, personal glorification or prowess is of no importance : lines of demarcation cease to exist.

Once a framework is provided with the various therapeutic disciplines of medicine, nursing, social work, physiotherapy and occupational therapy and speech therapy, not to mention the indispensable close and integrated administrative and secretarial systems, one needs the grouting cement of continuity to link all together. There are not nearly enough, nor indeed is the permitted complement enough to provide sufficient trained people to do all that is necessary. It has already been indicated how impossible it is to maintain all the links and all the many threads that are continually weaving and interweaving about each patient, and situation, coming into contact with the department. Links have to be forged and continuity maintained horizontally and vertically. How useless to coax back the patient's own confidence in his own capabilities, to walk or dress or to speak one day, and then not be able to reinforce this again for a considerable period. The absurdity of this kind of situation has been with us for many years of staff shortage.

Some four years ago it was felt that positive action would have to be taken to relieve the situation. People must be found who could provide the continuity needed. Many suggestions were made and many ideas discarded. There did not seem to be any category of staff within the hospital service whose function fitted the need of our patients for a true continuity maintainer. In the past, whenever there has been some sort of a gap in the service to hospital patients, it has been filled automatically, without thought or complaint, by the nursing staff. The decimation in their ranks has shown up all sorts of inadequacies in service that have lain totally submerged and unrecognised. Consequent upon the changing approach to illness, there has been a change in the use of the hospital bed, which is now only used either for sleeping in or as a clinical work bench. This has meant an entirely different pattern of life in the hospital ward. Patients are no longer analogous to the aged Thurber cat that lay in bed all day, following its owner round with its eyes and never moving.

We considered that there was a tremendous reservoir of goodwill in the community and that the spirit of service was just as great today as it has ever been. Could we find voluntary workers in sufficient numbers and with sufficient regularity to fill the gaps? A small pilot experiment soon answered this query. We found that although there was goodwill, the people we most needed could not manage just to *give* their services; they also needed some financial reward—firstly for the money itself, but also because the factor of having gainful employment conferred a certain feeling of confidence in their own capabilities.

Our Administrator searched around until he found a category in the welfare authority's domain called "an attendant on the aged and infirm" and he introduced this into our unit. The main purpose of this was that these people could, as a category, be under his control and not assigned to one discipline only, and by this means they could fulfil the inter-disciplinary requirements and be multi-functional. In the past it had been found, for instance, that nursing auxiliaries were necessarily attached to the matron and were therefore freely interchangeable about the hospital, and in any case were limited to nursing duties. Physiotherapy or occupational aides had the same limitations of function. Having found a category, and thus ensuring a pay packet, an advertisement was put in the local press, asking for part time help from people of goodwill and commonsense to help elderly, disabled patients regain their independence. There were 36 applications and from them one was chosen or, in a sense, was self-selected by her own attitude and approach.

We have had many aides since that time and we have found that their function is so unique that it is necessary that they should have a label in their own right, for they are not truly aides or auxiliaries or assistants or helps to any known disciplinary category. Their work is directly patient-centred, and in whatever direction the patient's need for support lies, they try to give it. They help to re-enable people to live again as sentient sophisticated adults and it was for this reason we coined the word 're-ablist'.

They have come in all shapes and sizes, from an ex-policewoman and a teacher of ceramics and art to housewives and mothers with no training except the very fine one involved in the running of a household and the bringing up of children.

At first we felt that the work must be fitted into some sort of career structure so that there would be the satisfaction of promotion and advancement and also, if it were national, there could be transference to other hospitals at the same grade for those who moved. But experience has suggested that there is a possibility that a career structure would tend to destroy the whole delicate balance, and would indeed be an invitation for infiltration by that bedeviller of so many disciplines—authoritarianism. It appears on present showing that just as the reablists fill a very great need in our framework, the framework itself is of value to them.

The strange condition which, for want of a better terminology, one could call the 'married woman syndrome' is a very real thing. The lack of confidence in her own capabilities of the woman who has been immured at home with her children for some years and fears that she is out of date and out of touch and who has no yardstick against which to measure herself as a marketable proposition. The role of reablist is ideally suited for her needs. All she requires is a genuine interest in people, a sound physical constitution, commonsense and a strong stomach and it is amazing how, after about a month's in-service training, the woman who has only committed herself cautiously to doing two or three hours a week is eagerly doing much more and enjoying it.

There has to be considerable flexibility on both sides with regard to hours. The principle firmly adhered to on our side, that school holidays, family illness and domestic crises take precedence and priority, has had the astonishing result that rarely do the reablists have to lose much time over these matters. Husbands, mothers and in-laws have been on our side too and cheerfully fill in, so allowing the reablists to carry on as normally possible. One husband was reported as saying, when his wife offered to give up work following his promotion, "Not on your life. You have not been as happy or as healthy for years as you have been since doing this job". Without a career structure, the life-span of a reablist seems to be, on average, about two years and then, confident in her own ability, she goes on to other things.

The wealth of experience reablists bring to the Unit, the variety of their personalities and their steadfastness has to be experienced to be understood.

The introduction of the reablist has done more to forge outside links with the community at large and to re-personalise the hospital existence of the patient than any other development in the Unit, and one hopes that in time we will gain authority to extend the work. This will not be easy as our Administrator has already been taken to task for this unorthodoxy and told from Ministry levels that such appointments must cease. As the Ministry has not indicated any alternative category, it is difficult to visualise where we go from there. One appreciates the desire of the Ministry that there should not be a proliferation of personnel categories within the Service. But how much more welcome would be a sign from on high of appreciation that work is being done and efforts being made to break the vicious circle of fewer staff and diminishing finances coping with tougher and more complex patient problems. How refreshing and relieving it would be to the workers in the arena if the planners from above actually defined the problems, discussed the remedies and supported us with all the power and resources at their command to provide the solutions. Awareness of the rapidly changing circumstances that engulf the front line worker seems to take an unconscionable age to penetrate back to the headquarters staff. By the time awareness comes, the opportune moment for action has often passed.

What shall we do then? Shut up shop altogether or concentrate on the recommendations made by T. D. Hunter[2] in his article on "New View of the Hospital—A Centre of Social Health":

"The hospital system needs to be radically re-structured.

1) Instead of being a mere 'supporting' service, the hospital must concentrate on becoming the dynamic centre of the socio-medical services and the active sponsor of preventive health work in the community.

2) It must provide comprehensive care and it must be democratically organised, i.e. organised on group lines rather than on individualistic or hierarchical lines. It should be patient-centred—planned not as a factory but as a total treatment hospital, as a therapeutic community, the varying types and gradations of patient care being provided within a single continuum of socio-medical knowledge. Especially is it important that the professional staff of the hospital, whether lay or specialised, should all have shared a basic training in the social sciences.

3) It must also function as a centre of positive health. It must aim at being a re-educative and regenerative force, exploiting to the full its links with, and its influence upon, the community. The hospital of tomorrow will have a new dimension; it will be a creator of values, a positive source of life norms and an active centre of humanism, of social solidarity. It will be a giver as well as a saver of life.

We must use it as a positive instrument of social reconstruction.

If we fail to take account of these propositions, we shall not build hospitals for tomorrow but, at best, for today. And, when tomorrow comes, today will already be yesterday."

"All that is needed for the triumph of evil is that good men do nothing".
Edmund Burke

References

1. Binks, F. Allen. (1968). *Brit. Med. J.*, **i,** 269-74.
2. Hunter, T. D. (1963). *Lancet,* **ii,** 933-35.

London, December 1967

Chapter Fourteen

LATER COMMUNICATION

Running throughout the last thirteen chapters is the theme of communication. Not everyone, perhaps, has discerned this but to me, re-reading the text after the passage of time, it is very apparent.

Perhaps the reason is not far to seek, for I was conscious from the day of publication that the charming little diagrams on *page 18,* on basic personal independence, were incomplete. For there are six basic needs, not five. The sixth is not the last nor the least, it is a primary need for a human being, it is the need to be able to communicate unaided.

The omission may have been fortuitous, as visually it would have set my artist a problem! On *page 86* I emphasised this need to communicate being of paramount importance where there is a case of speech difficulty, but this is not the only aspect of communication that is so vital.

Mention was made of the need for free communication between team workers, with patients and relatives, with the outside world of the community, and with other tiers of hierarchy in that conglomerate structure, the National Health Service. There is so much to this business of communication in our modern society. It is not just the method of communication and the varying techniques that are important, but also the content of the communication and the tuning of both the receptor and imparting mechanisms that can make or mar.

By one of those strange coincidences of which life is made, the publication of the first edition coincided with the publication of the first Green Paper,[1] and also the ministerial findings with regard to the questions raised in the first part of *Sans Everything*. While the former delighted me, the latter seemed a disappointingly ostrich-like method of dealing with a serious and courageous expression of public alarm.

It is interesting to reflect, before leaving the subject of *Sans Everything,* that often the bitterest critics of the book were those who had never read it. Many very senior members of the profession—whilst quite prepared to discuss the book as the work of unbalanced people, causing untold harm to the sacred cause of recruitment and the reputation of the handfuls of devoted workers in the field—were often exceedingly embarrassed when asked their opinion of the second part of the book *Some Answers.* In this, concrete proposals were made for improving the psychiatric services. Usually it became apparent that the book had been dismissed on hearsay, for very few reports of the book mentioned its gallant and constructive attempts to help 'authority' to right the wrongs described.

There is little doubt in my mind that Mrs. Barbara Robb and her colleagues, by their publication of *Sans Everything,* did more to help speed up improvement in the medical services to the patients of this country than has been done since Florence Nightingale bombarded the authorities with her *Memoranda.*

Let us remember, however, something that Dr. Robert Kemp has drawn attention to recently with his excellent article on *Our Obsession With The Hospital*[2] that Miss Nightingale "was probably inspired in her efforts by the universal poverty, the appalling housing and hygiene and the resultant mass of infection and deprivational disease". With our elderly today we are still faced by housing difficulties and deprivational disease, but as Dr. G. F. Adams has mentioned in another *multum in parvo* article : "mental confusion, disturbed behaviour and incontinence is the outstanding social and medical problem of our age, and this calls for readjustment of priorities and reallocation of resources . . . . Progress in medicine leaves wreckage in its wake and the community cannot afford either to concentrate these services too much on cure at the expense of care, least of all in our hospitals".

The first Green Paper (1968) seemed like an answer to my plea that the planners on high should actually define the problems, discuss the remedies and support the workers in the front line with all the power and resources at their command in order to provide the solutions. There seemed to be a dawning of light.

Indeed there should have been. Kenneth Robinson stated in

his foreword that he had been discussing the proposals since July 1965 with the Long Term Study Group.

The main suggestion of having unified health authorities, instead of the cumbersome autonomous tripartite system (Executive Council for GPs, Local Health and Welfare Authority and Hospital Service) seemed manna from heaven to us. We looked forward gladly to its instrumentation in a White Paper. Doubtless there would be many teething troubles, but the logic seemed irrefutable and it would do away with many of the problems we were meeting, which were not only wasteful of time and money but were also undermining patient and staff morale.

Of course, more important than any legislation are communication and personality—the personalities of the professionals, the patients and the neighbours. Also important are the need for constructive thought and the need for community action.

Already, without implementation of the Green Paper, we are aware of the first tender shoots of real community health teams springing up. We have several very productive ones round us. A small number of previously single-handed general practitioners have come together in group practices in purposely-constructed premises. They then gladly avail themselves of the proffered attachment from the local authorities of health visitors and home nurses, based on the practice premises and dealing with the practice patients, regardless of the various boundaries that previously formed iron curtains.

Intellectually we have seen much alteration in the content of our work and the type of referrals coming from such practices. Intellectually, because statistically, we have never found an opportunity to follow up the impressions by cold research. At one time we hoped to do this when offered a research worker for any project we cared to name, but the cup slipped and our lips remain parched as far as this is concerned. Someday one hopes this will be done—namely by a retrospective check on the type and mode of referral from individual general practitioners and by comparing these with a similar number of referrals after the doctors have joint group practices with full paramedical ancillary attachments. As a cynical, hard-bitten doctor working in geriatrics for three-quarters of a professional life, I would like to pay tribute here to my colleagues in the community who had the foresight and courage to take this step, to sink their prized independence in the strength of close-knit teams. By this they have increased immeasurably their service to the community they serve. Indeed some practices, so enheartened by the change, are incorporating other ancillary helpers into their teams and one can foresee a time when there will be mini-health clinics dotted about the community and functioning where people really live and not at remote distances. The chiropodist and the dentist, the physiotherapist, speech therapist, the occupational therapist, the bathing attendant, perhaps even home helps—would it not be possible to deploy them from the mini-clinics?

One far-seeing County Medical Officer of Health, Dr. I. A. MacDougall of Hampshire[3], is already advocating the attachment of home helps to group practices. He is a whole-hearted advocate for the Community Health Team and he estimates that the cost of looking after a patient in a hospital in his area averages out at £50 per week. The same patient looked after at home by the domiciliary team—allowing for a full-time residential home help (who would seldom be required), a daily half-hour visit by a district nurse and such visits as necessary by the doctor—would only cost about £18 per week. So this is an economically attractive goal quite apart from the humane aspects.

Given this happy state of affairs, the existing health and welfare clinic buildings could be utilised for training and community centres—in-service training for the professionals before and during attachment to the group practices and community day centres for the young, the handicapped, the elderly and any section of the community who need support and purposive occupation during the day. Such support could well reduce the need for permanent institutionalisation very considerably.

These ideas may seem impracticable administratively, but it is only by improvisation and trial and error that solutions will come. Traditional methods have not brought much relief to date. There ought to be experiment, flexibility and evaluation in order at least to provide an alternative to the modern white elephant in the National Health Service—the hospital. This last seems to be dying slowly, strangled by sheer size, weight and a greedy appetite for staff and funds which seems insatiable.

Post publication, I received an avalanche of letters from laymen, who had seen the press reports and then read the book. Apart from the odd letter or two from cranks, grinding their own particular axes, without exception these letters corroborated my thoughts and added fresh illustrations from their own experience. Not unnaturally there was no official comment and, alarmingly, very little comment from my medical colleagues unless they too happened to be working in the geriatric field. After a few months, however, in my turn I met embarrassment, but in a rather unexpected form. Lay-people who had read the book would ask what had happened. At first I was puzzled. What had happened about what? Well, had there been any action from 'the authorities' to put right some of the anomalies I had written about? Surely things must be different?

How can one explain to people not steeped and versed in the philistinism of traditional medical thought that a book such as mine, a mere worm's eye view of the monolithic structure, would have little more effect than a summer breeze rustling along the corridors of power. In this Erebus-like system where 'disposal' of people is accepted linguistic currency, where scholarly reports of official working parties make little impact, and Doreen Norton's ***Hospital of the Long-Stay Patient***[4] **and Peter Townsend's** ***The Last*** *Refuge,*[5] disappear without even leaving a worried mark, why should frail bleatings from one small corner of the juggernaut hope to produce response?

But let us be fair. Things have happened recently. There has been a record crop of official reports produced, advocating reform of the whole system. Each report published seems a masterpiece of judicious thought and each mentions that its suggestions and findings may need to be modified in the light of the other reports still to be published.

One's brain and mind reel from the plethora of reports, and yet what effect have they had, why is it that none of these outpourings appears to touch the collective medical conscience or alter by more than a perceptible degree the traditional ways of conduct?

One of the foremost of the official reports was called *First Report of the Joint Working Party on the Organisation of Medical Work in Hospitals.*[6] On its cover it had a clever little symbolic

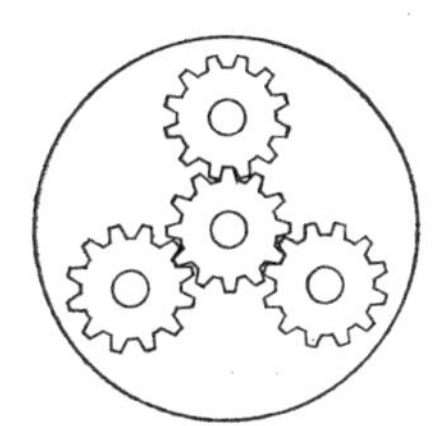

device and so came to be known rather endearingly by the title of the Cogwheel Report. This I suspect to have been the intention of astute members of the working party. Cogwheel is probably a masterpiece for all time—one can pick out of its context pure, shimmering, gold nuggets of commonsense cushioned delicately in beds of polite silken words, cajoling a change of heart and mind and thought from us tradition-bound doctors in all walks of life.

In mellifluous phrase it says virtually—doctors, for goodness' sake stop behaving in such individual and megalomaniac ways! Times have altered, the country and the Health Service need a different sort of doctor. The doctor must become one of a strong united team serving the community and become part of the community around him, he must no longer be a God-like individualist expecting all to acquiesce in his way of thinking and doing. He has to learn to communicate, co-operate and co-ordinate.

Cogwheel said in its preface: "Hospitals have tended to work in isolation from other parts of the community health services . . ."

"The stay of a patient in hospital is however only one event in the disease sequence. Hospitals may be involved in the care of patients before admission . . . . and after discharge with follow-up or rehabilitation." Cogwheel considered that there was "no doubt that the efficiency of the hospital service in the future depends upon the radical revision of traditional methods of organising medical work in hospital. This process must be the outcome of local consideration and conviction rather than the imposition of detailed methods arbitrarily defined centrally."

"The identifications of problems within the complex of services and a fresh approach to them can bring about improvement *without awaiting reform of the administrative structure.*" The italics are mine.

Too true. The cogwheels unfortunately are only too symbolic. Like the mills of God they seem to grind slowly and exceeding small. The reports seem to come out and churn round each other delicately, defining, suggesting, hinting, but never directing. The cogs mesh and unmesh but no results seem to come.

Cogwheel 1967, the first Green Paper 1968, then the Williams, Seebohm, Maud, Todd and Aves reports and probably many more—all these are blueprints of cogent reasoning, produced after years of intensive deliberation and conscientious questioning of hosts of people from a very wide cross-section of those engaged in health and welfare services in this country. How many of these reports have you, the reader, heard about and, better still, how many of them have you read? Yet all have a vital bearing on our day-to-day life as citizens.

Now with a flourish of trumpets comes the long-heralded new-look Green Paper, price 25 new pence. At last we think unification has arrived and the consumer is to receive a comprehensive service emanating from one light source, the Health Board. All the strange anomalies and devious 'proper' channels and side routes will become one clear highway. Never need things happen again in the way they did to Miss Benbow.

Yes, Miss Benbow. Let us look at Miss Benbow's story and see whether the recommendations now being made would have smoothed her path if they had then been in force.

Miss Benbow spent twenty-five months with us in our ward in the district hospital. At the then current £35 a week, that works out at £3,500 which is quite a sum.

In age Miss Benbow is two years older than the year and she was only a stripling (to us) of 69 when her initial referral came. The referral came from one of our medical officer of health colleagues, which was unusual. He had been asked by his team to see Miss Benbow and help to decide on her future management, as they felt she had got beyond the facilities they could offer in the way of home support. The MOH was in a quandary too, for Miss Benbow was as bright as a button and determinedly wishing to remain at home. He could not decide whether this was feasible, by installing hoists and other paraphernalia, or whether she could be managed in one of his welfare home beds or whether hospital would be best. She was very incontinent but she said this was unnecessary and only due to lack of opportunity and facility for getting to the lavatory, but the doctor was dubious. We agreed to visit and give an opinion, and the general practitioner added his pleas for speedy help, for the patient was developing pressure sores and the supporting neighbours were giving up.

As usual the story reaches back many years. Occasionally one wonders how Henry Ford made his money if he really thought "history is bunk". History is the stuff of which we are made and, as so invariably happens, Miss Benbow's full history did not become completely known until long after she came to us; even now fresh parts of the jigsaw keep turning up. The key pieces are as follows:

Miss Benbow had been a shop assistant, and lived with her parents and looked after them until their deaths—mother at 80 and father later at 85. Then she went to live with her brother, prudently at the same time putting her name down on the council housing list for a small flat.

In 1961 she developed what she thought to be chilblains on her left toes and later she noticed a painful swelling behind the knee of the same leg. Two months' home treatment failed to help, the leg became much worse and she was admitted to the small general hospital H near her home. This hospital boasted close connections with a famous teaching hospital X. She was soon transferred to X Hospital which dealt admirably with her gangrenous leg, which had to be amputated at the thigh, and *pari passu* the diabetes she was found to have.

The Limb-fitting Centre R, again some distance away, provided her with a pylon and eventually an artificial leg, and Miss Benbow retraced her steps via H Hospital to home. Via H Hospital, she also received two wheelchairs, one a folding one in which she could be pushed out and about and the other a rigid self-propelling one. This latter was a commode-type and an open one at that without any covering seat, but she required this because the lavatory was upstairs and she could not then negotiate stairs.

From home Miss Benbow attended a Physical Therapy Centre T and soon she had made a marvellous return to personal independence on her new full-length leg and supporting wooden crutches. She went out shopping and even helped a busy professional woman by minding her children.

Meantime she kept her follow-up appointments at two or three monthly intervals at the distant X Hospital where obviously they were very proud of her. She needed readmission there in the winter of that year when her right leg also appeared to be in jeopardy.

The next milestone was a pleasant one, she was offered a new ground-floor flat in a big new block in a close of new dwellings. The flat had a small bathroom, combining bath, basin and lavatory, a kitchen and a bed-sitting room, but no central heating or warden support. A further drawback was that it was some distance from the shops and though there was a fairly high density population in a small compass, there was no public telephone or pillar-box in the close. A strange planning omission but far from infrequent in new developments, one notices—again showing the need for communication, this time ironically, between the country's main channel of communication, the Post Office, and local authority housing departments. These are points one bemoans time and time again, but soon mayhap these things will be included as fundamental in community housing plans of this kind.

Miss Benbow seemed to manage well in her new flat until once more in the winter her right foot gave trouble and she had to be admitted to X Hospital yet again to have her toenail removed and the underlying infection drained. This was a much shorter admission of only a few weeks.

For two years all went well except there were alarms and excursions with regard to her left eye which entailed her attending two different hospital eye departments. Eventually the eye had to be removed as an emergency and six months later, just as she was recovering from this blow, she had a stroke, paralysing her left side.

Once more she went through the rigmarole of ping-ponging from one hospital to another, but despite this it was noted by a physiotherapist that though she was very lively and plucky, she did tend to take her disabilities too lightly! A new limb prosthesis was ordered, because the stroke had affected the fitting of the old one, but in each hospital efforts were made to make Miss Benbow realise that she could no longer manage independently in her own flat, alone.

The arguments could not have been convincing enough, for Miss Benbow, one gathers, took her own discharge and went home. She had good neighbours, a brother near, a home nurse once a week to help her bath, and a home help three times a week. Consequently it was fifteen months before she was referred to us and she had to be referred to us, of course, because by her own intransigent attitude she had forfeited the concern of her own local general hospital H and the teaching hospital X. They were able to refuse to have anything further to do with her—she was now geriatric and it had to be the geographically distant and despised geriatric department from whom help was sought.

One can only piece together what must have happened in the intervening fifteen months by guesswork and from chance remarks made by others involved, for from Miss Benbow little came. Her fury and resentment and humiliation were so profound at coming to what seemed to her an alien and second class hospital that they clouded and coloured the relationship of all who came into contact with her after admission. She was terrified of having to lose her remaining leg which was ulcerated and which also had a deep pressure sore on the heel. She probably felt that she was now institutionalised for good. I was soon sent roundly about my business and realised that it would be better to let those who were more acceptable deal with her and not exacerbate the situation further. There were several misapprehensions and misconceptions about Miss Benbow from the beginning, for the whole business had been snarled and be-fogged by the conflicting stories circulating and Miss Benbow had been no great help in clarifying matters.

My colleague who had seen her at home had been puzzled how she had managed so long on her own, as her condition was truly appalling. She had obviously spent a prolonged period sitting day and night on the open commode wheelchair which, as he had noted, was designed for two-arm propulsion and she had had to use it one-handedly. She told him that after two falls from the chair, whilst trying to get herself a meal, she had abandoned attempts to use the kitchen at all.

Another difficulty had been the lavatory, for she could not get into the bathroom without help and, after reduction of home help time from thrice to once weekly, her brother's move away from the area and the illness of supporting neighbours, she had supposedly become incontinent.

When she arrived in hospital her bellicose attitude created an entirely false impression of her personality. Her chair followed her and its filthy condition was tangible evidence of the deplorable state into which she had fallen. She sat in her rather dark corner of the ward, her artificial leg stuck in the corner behind her, one opaque lens in her spectacles and her grim expression giving her a somewhat malevolent appearance. Further attempts to help her drew forth pungent bitter comparisons between the sublime X Hospital of hallowed and revered memory and our inadequate facilities and attenuated staffing complement.

The deep pressure sore on her heel and the very precarious state of circulation in her good leg meant that little could be done in the way of active remobilisation towards weight-bearing. It took eleven months before the heel was soundly healed and it was safe for her to weight-bear once more. In the interim period we had not been totally inactive on her behalf and a folding one-handed self-propelling non-commode wheelchair had been ordered, and the noisome and repellent one returned.

Soon the sun began to peep out from behind the black cloud and though Miss Benbow would not join in with any group activity and remained glued to her corner, she was doing more and more and was learning to transfer from bed to chair without needing too much help.

There was no question of her learning to transfer from wheelchair to lavatory as our ward lavatory is so designed as to make it impossible for a person in a wheelchair with footrests on to obtain entrance. Endeavours were made to help with these problems by taking her down to the Further Activity Centre to practise. Even this was doomed to failure, something or somebody there upset her *amour-propre* and she refused to make the trip again after a time.

She just clamoured to get home. Unfortunately her general demeanour affected some of our staff in the same way it had at H and X hospitals. They reckoned she was unrealistic and that with her amount of disability she could never manage again at home. To still her clamour, arrangements were made to take her to meet the welfare officer for the handicapped at her flat so that she could be assessed in consultation. The welfare officer knew her well and had tried previously to get her to apply for residential care.

Now the other cause for her dependency became apparent—the bathroom door in her flat was only twenty-five inches wide and the average adult wheelchair width was at least twenty-five inches. So Miss Benbow had not only been handicapped by the wrong type of wheelchair, but there had never been the remotest chance of her getting her rigid self-propelling chair into the bathroom. Therefore she had always needed help to get her leg on, so that she could walk into the bathroom. Once there, a raised lavatory seat had enabled her to be independent but the hazards were truly formidable.

After this visit, professional controversy raged, and ranged from suggestions for taking off the bathroom door, knocking down the wall, to putting in parallel bars to enable the patient to walk in. The first move seemed obvious and that was to request help from the Ministry's technical officer with regard to the chair. The head technical officer came and subsequently a specially modified chair that would both take Miss Benbow's bulk and go through the narrow bathroom doorway.

Now more controversy raged about the next move. What adaptations should the Welfare Department be asked to arrange and was the inevitable expense to public funds justified? A number of people felt that the patient was completely non-viable at home.

At this point Miss Benbow refused to make any more trips home, nor would she go down to the Further Activity Centre if the welfare officers came to see her. A classic picture of self-fulfilling prophecy, she was an unrealistic, unco-operative person and, lo and behold, here she was behaving in an unrealistic, unco-operative way! To Miss Benbow it was all such stuff and nonsense that she turned her chair round to face the wall and presented her back to the ward and to visitors.

This was ideal. One of the most important factors for the future hinged on whether she could reverse her wheelchair out of her bathroom there being no room in there to turn it. She was asked to demonstrate this to the visiting welfare officers and in order to maintain a steady flow of soothing patter and so prevent the emergence of any excoriating remark from Miss Benbow, she was asked what adaptations she thought were necessary to make her independent at home?

Unhappy day! There it was again, the professional omnipotence that can be the malignant familiar of us all, however hard we try. This was the first time, seemingly, anyone had asked the patient! She said she only needed one straight, stout wall-bar by the lavatory and she could manage completely independently.

We were all so dumbfounded that, smug with her success, she deigned to demonstrate, using the handrail in the corridor as the proposed support and a commode positioned to double as the lavatory at home. Sure enough without an atom of assistance, except to stabilize the commode, she pivoted smoothly from wheelchair to 'lavatory'—using only the wall-bar to help. As this was at the wrong height and of the wrong dimension for her impaired grip it was quite a remarkable feat.

To the hospital team, all now seemed to be a straightforward mechanical transaction that would soon be accomplished. Details of height, type, position and size of rail were supplied to the Welfare Department and that would be that.

It took six months.

Firstly it had to go before a Committee, then to the Housing Department for permission to do structural alterations. The architect had to visit and make plans, the job then had to be put out to tender; tenders had to come in and be vetted and passed, and the work then had to be carried out. As it was a partition wall, there were certain difficulties. The job was going to cost £17 and this was felt to be excessive and so the months dragged on.

This strange economic extravaganza weighed on our minds. One week's stay in hospital was the equivalent of two wall-bars at £17 a time. How many wall-bars could one install for £840, which was the cost to the community to keep Miss Benbow in hospital for six months?

Then the bright day dawned. A triumphant telephone call told us the bar was installed. When was Miss Benbow to be discharged home? Some sixth sense bade us hasten slowly and arrange an afternoon visit home first, plus Miss Benbow and wheelchair. This took a little time to organise as she lived a long way from the hospital. A time was agreed upon and the necessary cars set out. Unhappily it was one of the coldest days of the season and a Siberian wind whistled through the Close. Miss Benbow, always a poor traveller, vomited all the way to the flat. To ease her the car windows had to be kept opened and the heater turned off. Fortunately Miss Benbow ignores cold but the three team members in the car with her almost had to be chipped out at the other end. The key left with her was the wrong one and the welfare officer, with the right one, was delayed for half an hour.

A kind neighbour took pity on the group and warmed the team with tea and sympathy, but Miss Benbow with clenched teeth refused to budge from the car. Eventually the front door was unlocked and the convoy entered the freezing flat. Miss Benbow directed the gas to be turned on and the solitary gas-fire lit and then the rail was inspected.

The culminating horror—the rail was totally inadequate! With the best intentions in order to make a neat job and to ensure stability the rail had been sunk tidily into a recess of the wall, well out of Miss Benbow's reach for functional use. No reference had been made to us of this change of position at any time so that its ineffectiveness could have been explained. Feelings ran high. No warmth of customary camaraderie flowed between hospital and welfare team. All repaired miserably and bleakly home, or in Miss Benbow's case back to the hospital.

Two more months went by and many telephone calls and close shaves with further inadequate fixtures, and then again all was ready. At least the cold weather had departed. Miss Benbow refused a further trial run, she would only go home permanently now. And this, to cut an interminable story short, is what happened and she has now been there for over a year, safely and very happily, and furthermore it transpires that, as a housekeeper, she is a perfectionist and all is spotless.

This despite the trials of a sink with taps too high and cupboards out of her reach (she will not allow any alterations in her kitchen). To see her light her only form of heating, her gas fire, is enough to frighten the stoutest heart. Being one-handed she has to lean down, turn on the gas, then drop a lighted match into the fire, for the automatic lighting mechanism needs two hands and is at the bottom. Recently the natural gas came to her area and equipment has been exchanged. Unfortunately no one suggested she should have one of the fires with top controls, and her hazardous fire lighting ritual continued. Further communication, coincidentally at a Relatives' Conference with the natural gas organisers, has speeded rectification.

I have recounted the Benbow chronicle at some length. I could quote yet another from a different welfare authority where, forewarned by Miss Benbow's difficulties, we alerted the housing and welfare departments well in advance. Consequently they were on their mettle and 'rushed' through the provision of grab rails at strategic points in a matter of two months. Let us consider whether, under the new design outlined in the 1970 White Paper,[7] things would have happened more expeditiously and whether by 'unification' under an Area Health Board an intended discharge like this would have progressed smoothly forward and thus saved the community some £3,000 at least.

In fact, of course, it would have made no difference. For the alterations needed and the agencies involved all lay in the area of the local authority service—the social and welfare officers, the architect and surveyor, the housing department, the authorising council committee, even the home help and meals-on-wheels and good neighbour schemes. None of these would have been produced any faster under the new formula. Only the provision of the home nurse would have been an Area Health Board concern and there is rarely difficulty about this at any time now.

What is more important than any legislation is the need for direct communication between the people involved in situations such as this. More important too are the personalities of the patient, professionals, the relatives and neighbours and the need for constructive thought and action all the way through. Neither Miss Benbow's fifteen months' battle at home nor her subsequent twenty-five months' stay with us would have been necessary, if more thought had gone into her original discharge from H Hospital after the stroke. This need never have been the corrosive affair it became, if someone had thought to supply her with a wheelchair suited to her particular needs. Even measuring the bathroom door would have helped. If a new wheelchair had been ordered, these points would have been covered because the application form questions the need for two or one-handed propulsion and also asks for the width of the narrowest doorway that has to be negotiated.

We learnt recently that purpose-built housing for the elderly is still being designed with bathroom doors only twenty-five inches wide, which seems a pity as more disabled people are being assisted to live at home. As Cogwheel said in 1967:

> "Recognition of the need for continuity of care and integration of the constituent services, including the preventive services of the local authority, is widespread and seems at variance with the continuance of administrative divisions within the National Health Service."
>
> "The present arrangements for integrating 'care'—including diagnosis, treatment and after-care—are inadequate."
>
> "The organisation of medical care in this country on a national basis, with increasing emphasis on the concept that the total medical care of the patient requires the integrated co-operation of services inside and outside hospital, [is more vital] now than ever before . . . .".
>
> "Problems of management proliferate in an organisation with many branches, many functions, and many specialities. Opportunities for failure of communication abound in such situations."

Soon will come official pronouncement on the Seebohm Report 1969 and it would seem to me that the main future schism in the service is likely to come if the recommendations made in the Seebohm Report are accepted. That the Seebohm Committee ever came to be needed, doctors can only blame themselves and their lack of perception and concern for the social implications and results associated with illness.

Social workers, smarting under years of seeming servitude and professional frustration, have revolted and now plan to be autonomous and quite separate from the medical fraternity. Understandable though this is, as far as professional disciplinary pride is concerned, it is hard to reconcile this approach when seen from the patients' or, in social work terminology, the clients' viewpoint. For Seebohm recommendations reduced to primitive fact constitute a plea for all types and conditions of social workers to unite in autarchy and be free for ever from medical bondage.

One has a vision of the medical forces of the country coalescing on one side and the social forces on the other and like a great

Red Sea dividing and rolling back, with the anxious patient-client walking along the divide, hoping no doubt to reach safety without being engulfed from either side or, worse, becoming a storm-tossed cork in the middle.

These are no idle musings. The Annual Report of the powerful Central Health Services Council has condemned the proposals in the Seebohm Report that medical social work should be separated. They suggest that this would be administratively disastrous and would be to the great disadvantage of the patient. If we do not, as a community, wake up to the legislative build-up around us, we seem likely to be crushed into stunned acquiescence in the not too distant future.

Margaret Blenkner[8], an American social worker, tells the story of an old man applying for admission to an apartment house for older people, opened by a social agency for which she was directing a study of a model programme of services to the ageing. They gave him the works in the way of study and diagnosis. The caseworker interviewed him, the public health nurse visited him, a physician examined him. He made a trial visit to the apartment house, he met and talked with house staff and residents. They held innumerable staff conferences about him. They had a psychiatric consultation and altogether it was a glorious inter-disciplinary experience in psychobiosocial diagnosis for all—except the old man. After several weeks, they concluded their deliberations and decided he was a proper candidate for residence in the house. He was called in and the service director, exuding the warmth of the professional offering a tangible reward for good client performance, informed him of their decision. Puzzled by his somewhat flat response, she asked, "Aren't you pleased?"

"I guess so," the old man sighed. Then with rising inflection, "But that was a helluva lot to go through just to rent a room!"

An amusing story and because of the slight trans-Atlantic twist our laugh can be a shade patronising. But should it be? These things are happening to us here in this United Kingdom now. Our hospitals are becoming more and more like technical factories 'turning-over' cases. Those who cannot be compressed or expanded to fit the scientific Procrustean hospital bed are then deemed social misfits or geriatric problems and, willy-nilly, are extruded as acute bed-blocking pariahs, this extrusive process being accomplished by subtle moral blackmail, which should be a disgrace to professional conscience.

Strong words? No words are too strong to describe some of the pressures and manoeuvres that are used in the effort to 'dispose' of the socially and clinically unprepossessing—the person who has the temerity to remain in a general medical or surgical bed once his period of interestingness has finished.

Great play is made of the need to free scarce beds in order to do dramatic deeds of Kildare-daring, to save important young wage-earning lives. The cry of hospital bed shortage has been going on so long that the medical professions and the public at large have been well brainwashed into honestly believing that, as there is such an overall shortage, seriously ill people are being kept out of hospital because old people are occupying beds needlessly.

Cogwheel 1967 mentioned that administrators, and others, often tend to give undue weight to bed occupancy figures. As a result, patients may occasionally be kept in hospital for longer than necessary, regardless of the adverse effect on turnover and actual bed use, and with no consideration for the desire of the patient to return home.

The sophisticated methods of the Hospital Activity Analysis have enabled Professor D. J. Newell of the Medical Care Research Unit of Newcastle University[9] to draw the interesting conclusion that whatever the shortages of facilities in the Health Service they cannot now be attributed to a national shortage of beds.

"Despite a 10 per cent reduction in the availability of hospital beds per head of population in the last ten years, the bed occupancy rate has in fact fallen from 87 to 84 per cent. Where one in seven beds was empty ten years ago, now one in six is empty.

"The beds may be in the wrong places, allocated to the wrong uses, understaffed or without other essential facilities, but on an average day there 75,000 beds empty in the country." A truly staggering and sobering thought!

This being so, how can we account for the tremendous pressure put on the relatives of elderly patients to take them out of the hospital long before they are independent, in order to make way for the mythical, needy young person. Indeed, pressure is often put on the patient himself.

Frequently an elderly sick person comes into hospital because conditions at home are not suitable for him to be supported there. What amazing double-think has to occur to suggest return to such conditions before complete return to personal independence has been achieved. What can concerned relatives and humbled old people do under such circumstances but accept the list of nursing homes which is proffered as an alternative, and scurry round to find a vacancy in the one matching most nearly not the patient's need but his pocket's depth?

The recent Dan Mason report, *Home from Hospital,* devotes a chapter to thumbnail sketches of the needs of eighteen out of the 533 patients studied. The eighteen were taken as examples of the worst instances of hardship encountered and was an indictment of the callous lack of thought that can occur when discharging people from hospital. The examples were not all amongst the elderly either. From our own experiences, we know that the examples quoted were far from extraordinary.

In recent years there seems to have been a veritable mushrooming of homes for the elderly and ones already established have expanded and the charges have rocketed. No figures or research seem to be available on the use of private nursing homes to camouflage this obnoxious and flagrant piece of medical legerdemain, for there is no overall shortage of hospital beds, only an artificially produced shortage for those who are deemed irremediable.

Paradoxically the free National Health Service (or almost free for, ironically, the State pensioner surrenders £2 of his weekly pension after he has been in hospital eight weeks and £4 after a year and he is the only hospital user to be mulcted involuntarily in this way) seems to have boosted the use and growth of the commercial nursing home for custodial purposes, for there is no statutory institute of imperative relegation left in this country apart from prison.

The workhouse disappeared with the advent of the National Health Service in 1948. The mental hospitals remained as a bolthole until the mental health legislation in 1959. Until then the vast conurbations of mental hospitals, some containing over 2,000 beds, were tucked away out of the community's sight in the country. After 1948 they were the recipients of the dropouts from society and of the rejects from the more 'respectable' acute hospital systems.

Since 1959, the mental hospitals too have been permitted selectivity and the last stronghold of statutory carpet under which our unprepossessing people can be swept for 'disposal' has vanished.

When an opportunity arose in the autumn of 1969, I attempted to draw attention to this new phenomenon in an interview with a journalist. This interview was printed in February 1970 and it was a powerful piece of journalistic writing, part of a short series on the *Disposable Society*. The letters to the paper that followed were from the lay public caught in the traps that the article mentioned. Despite the coat-trailing, there was no comment from elsewhere.

In the article was quoted an incident in which I had recently been involved and which was one of a series that had particularly shocked my thrifty Scots blood. An elderly lady who had had a stroke was admitted to a big hospital. In a few weeks the relatives were told she was to be discharged as no more could be done for her and she was blocking a needed bed. She was not independent for her own needs or able to return to living alone. In the time available the son had only been able to find a vacancy in a nursing home in our area, which had been graciously pleased to accept her at the customary £35 per week. The bulk of this her family had to find as she had only her pension to live on. She had a room to herself and to all intents and purposes everything she needed, except a place in society and a purpose for living.

She became incontinent as people isolated, inactive and purposeless often do. Soon a urinary infection developed and the drugs used for its treatment produced a violent skin reaction. To stop her scratching herself to bits, she required considerable sedation and a special nurse night and day. This put up her fees by another £70 per week. Add to this basic £105, the extras for drugs, laundry, diet, *etc.*, and she soon had a bill of £120 per week. A weekly sum few families can sustain even in this affluent society and sure enough it was not long before help had to be sought from the statutory service. On this occasion our department was involved and I saw her on a visit.

Since that (to me) particularly shocking situation, a number of similar economic and human tangles have come our way and are continuing to do so in a steady trickle.

My concern is on two counts, leaving aside the emotional and humane issues. Firstly the growth of commercial nursing homes on this apparent scale can only be underpinned by having a National Health Service. The staff manning such homes are being trained in the NHS hospitals and then many of them leave the service to join nursing homes, or agencies, attracted by the vastly better salaries. When financial drought hits the patient and families, it is the statutory service that then has to underpin again, by readmitting the patient to hospital, usually in a much more inert and demoralised state than when discharged initially.

The second point is the contention that these situations should never have occurred in the first place. We are living in a Welfare State. If a person is unfit to live in a local authority residential home, then they must *ipso facto* still require hospital support. There can be no falling between the two stools into the grey crippling world of commercially orientated nursing homes, except by exercise of very personal choice. This cannot be Hobson's choice.

Exerting emotional blackmail to get old people out of hospital must be stopped. Charitable and voluntary societies could do a good deal to help and to educate reluctant and recalcitrant professional philistines by refusing to help subsidise such situations. They should only help with financial assistance those who have opted voluntarily and determinedly to use nursing homes despite all other statutory offers. Such people are becoming fewer in number as the older generation, unused to the Welfare State, gradually dies out.

In the interview with the journalist I suggested that the whole situation could be clarified if a test case was brought to trial, in an instance where an old person had been turned out of hospital and the relatives had been obliged to find a nursing home place more or less under duress, as the old person was not personally independent and the relatives were unable to support the situation at home.

Later Communication

In this country, relatives are still too dutiful and responsible to dream of going to law over matters such as this, though legally sons and daughters are no longer held responsible for their parents. The majority still accept responsibility as a moral duty, in those rare cases where there is little mutual esteem and affection.

The figures quoted in *Old People in Three Industrial Societies* make astonishing reading. Of the pensionable population in this country, 42 per cent live with sons or daughters (a higher figure than ever previously known). In the USA the figure is 27 per cent, and in Denmark 20 per cent. [In Sweden it is only 10 per cent.]

When this fact is coupled with the information that at any one time in this country there is never more than 6 per cent of the pensionable population in hospital or in old people's homes, one feels that containment of such problems as there are must be well within our administrative and economic power, if only the leadership and inclination was also there.

"It is darkest immediately under the candle."

Chinese Proverb

References

1. *The Administrative Structure of the Medical and Related Services in England and Wales.* HMSO, 1968.
2. Kemp, Robert. *Our Obsession With the Hospital.* British Journal of Hospital Medicine, November 1969.
3. MacDougall, I. A. *Developing the Community Health Team.* Health Trends. HMSO. July, 1970.
4. Norton, Doreen, *Hospitals of the Long-Stay Patient.* Pergamon Press. 1967.
5. Townsend, Peter. *The Last Refuge.* Routledge and Kegan Paul. 1962
6. *First Report of the Joint Working Party on the Organisation of Medical Work in Hospital.* HMSO. 1967.
7. *The Future Structure of the National Health Service.* HMSO. 1970.
8. Blenkner, Margaret. *The Dependencies of Old People.* Ed. Richard Kalish. Institute of Gerontology. University of Michigan. 1969.
9. Newell D. J. *Hospital Bed Usage.* British Journal of Hospital Medicine. June 1970.

Chapter Fifteen

STOP PRESS OR ENVOI

Even as the first edition came off the press a long expected and eagerly awaited local event occurred. An event that had been suggested and discussed for about two years before it happened and the actual date of happening had altered interminably, so that ultimately the area workers hardly knew it had come about. A geriatric ward of twenty beds was opened at Mount Vernon Hospital and a small region, namely the postal district of Pinner, was removed from our area of territorial responsibility. Our masters expected us to be much overjoyed at this relief and were puzzled and hurt at the lack of gratitude that we exhibited, but in the light of cold statistics it was only equivalent to removing a few straws from the load. Our overall population at risk is now 420,000, the over-65 population 48,000, so we should have 480 beds but still our overall bed complement remains the same.

Two other events have occurred also : *ie* two of the so precariously held annexes have finally folded. Oxhey Grove (*see Figure 3, page 12*) became structurally untenable and the patients were moved to a ward in West Hendon Hospital. This move was the culmination of many weary months of planning, administrative battle and rearguard action. The personal moral courage that is often required by people working in the geriatric field to face the combined pressures from other factions who perceive tidy, neat and cheap solutions to geriatric problems is something that can rarely be described.

It is to be recalled that in Oxhey Grove there was no lavatory available for the use of the 30 patients—the solitary one on the ground floor being accessible through the kitchen, the first floor one through the staff quarters. This placed certain constraints on the abilities of patients transferred to this annexe. Inevitably they had to be bed or chair bound people who would be unaware of this social deprivation. Consequently when as a substitute for these premises three wards in an isolation hospital were offered, it was not considered that many alterations would be required in order to make a 100 per cent improvement in the environment. For fever wards are by regulation large, airy, spacious places with wide spaces between the beds. The three wards were also, of course, isolated from each other with roadways between.

The geriatric team spent many long midnight hours trying to devise a way of welding together these three wards into a functional unit where integration, not isolation, could be aided. Eventually it was decided from Regional level that the two adjacent wards should be joined by a new structural infill, and the small third one left alone *pro tem*. The heating, electrical and plumbing facilities of the hospital were due for upgrading in any case—but when suggestions for doubling the bed complement were blocked by the mad geriatricians and insane demands for the provision of many more lavatories, wash-basins and bathing facilities were made, things really began to warm up.

I was privileged to be at the meeting organised to crush finally this insurrection of geriatric folly. Patiently the heavyweights from the Regional Board explained that one lavatory per five patients was the Regional Board figure. Patiently they pointed out that our patients' situation would be vastly improved by the mere move away from inadequate premises. Firmly our consultant riposted that where there were long-stay patients requiring maximum support, then the very best facilities, equipment and staff-ratio were required, not just the bare minimum.* He realised that one lavatory and wash-basin per person were unrealistic at that time but one lavatory to three patients was the minimum—plus the same fever bed-spacing, plus dining and day rooms, and so on. It was a strained meeting, many cross-currents of vested interest and emotion tensed the atmosphere and eventually the inevitable confrontation point was reached. One lone consultant stated firmly,

*Duncan Guthrie, Chairman of the Central Council for the Disabled, propounds this succinctly: "The importance of the environment increases in direct proportion to the amount of time that the occupant is obliged to spend in it."

"You can direct me to do this, but I will not undertake this responsibility voluntarily unless there is maximum upgrading of these wards to produce reasonably civilised standards." The day was won. The ward now has the requisite number of lavatories—a memorial to one of the many episodes of moral courage that are called for far too frequently in this 'civilised society'.

This was making the best of what was offered. In effect we now have a ward 100-yards long and, opening off, are day rooms. There is more privacy for the patients when in bed with bed-curtains drawn because there is reasonable space between the beds. However, the running of such a structure is a minor nightmare for the nursing staff unless there are many of them. Interestingly too, although the number of wash-basins requested has been provided, the actual placing of them makes them almost useless from the patients' point of view, as it is not possible to curtain them off for privacy in use.

Though in theory we had expected improvement in the general well-being of the patients, not one of us was prepared for the veritable transformation that occurred, once they had become accustomed to the move. People who for years had seemed beyond contact-recall responded almost like flowers opening in the sun. The opportunity to get from one room to another—albeit in a wheelchair—to get dressed and participate in group and individual activities wrought a real sea-change. This was all the more pleasing for-as-much-as many people had expected that only the *élite* of 'best' patients from the unit as a whole would be picked to occupy these plush premises. There had been some displeasure that all the most disabled people had been moved together. Our only regret was that we failed to take cine film of the before and after effect. Never has there been such a clear demonstration that if people are offered reasonable conditions in which to live, then they will live up to their maximum—not down to their minimum.

This then was heartening. We were well aware that in time and as the need for isolation hospital beds decreased, other wards at West Hendon Hospital would fall to our lot and inevitably other far-flung annexes would have to be closed willy-nilly, as it became increasingly more difficult to get staff replacements when long-serving faithfuls retired. Glebe House (the old country house one mile from the nearest bus stop) had struggled gallantly on from hand to mouth as far as adequate staffing went, ever since I had known it. Crisis after crisis was weathered by the devoted efforts of the permanent staff. Final collapse came, however, when not only were they many nursing and domestic staff down but there was no gardener-handyman either and the unhappy decision had to be made to move the patients urgently. This meant using another ward at West Hendon, doing only the minimum upgrading necessary to make it reasonably habitable.

All this has reduced the far-flung nature of the unit and shortened the lines of communication, but strangely has thrown a greater burden on a different echelon of staff. Very little was possible before in the way of activity because of limitations of space and facility. Now it is important that people should get up and dress for a purpose, other than just a meal and then a return to bed. All people do not respond to the same motivating forces and to provide a choice of interests and activity for both men and women—many severely handicapped—demands a great deal from our limited forces of occupational and physiotherapy staff, for the ranks of nursing staff have not been reinforced further and they are fully stretched already with their routine duties.

Now our reablists are truly coming into their own and we have been able to increase the complement modestly. This is a headache of co-ordination where two or three people, part-time, represent one unit of full-time reablist, but the value of their contribution to the integration of disparate isolated wards justifies all the headaches involved. They are the community coming in. They are the ordinary commonsense laymen with the different non-traditional outlook that we jaded, conditioned professionals need. The Green Paper mentions the need to foster local participation in the work of the hospitals. There is a musing as to "whether existing personnel can with further training undertake wider functions and whether new forms of generic training need be developed". The Secretary of State need look no further. In geriatric departments up and down the country, where necessity has been the mother of invention and sheer survival has depended on the development of many unusual forms of self-help, he will find numerous ideas that are worthy of further study and development. There is always a danger that new ideas are seized upon as the universal panacea for all problems without modifying or easing them into local context, so that one man's lifeline could easily strangle another drowning man, if ill-applied. In our own small complex we have seen reablists defeated by the attitude of the professional staff to them. The use of reablists must be purposeful, positive, constructive and welcomed by the professional staff. To use them purely as pairs of inferior hands and gap-stoppers will never lead to ease of relationship or recruitment.

Surely other changes must have occurred in two years? Surely if it is stated policy that half the beds of a geriatric unit should be in the district hospital, there must have been a great increase in the number allocated in the parent hospital? On paper, yes. On paper, we have ten more beds for women, as the previously named ten chronic surgical beds (the occupants of which we have supported clinically for some years in any case) are now officially allocated to us. So we now have officially forty-eight beds in the district hospital. Still our colleagues from the general side in the Group complain that their beds are filled with 'our' patients, but the rush to augment our bed complement with the obviously surplus 'acute' beds could be controlled easily by a blind, totally paralysed traffic warden! Unceasingly and unremittingly we are told we are not clearing our colleagues' blocked beds, therefore we are not doing our job. "Too long a sacrifice does make a stone of the heart." Perhaps, to mix our metaphors further, we are no longer able to see the wood for the trees. Certainly we seem totally unable to speak so that our colleagues can hear and understand. Where lies the breakdown in communication? Does it lie in the receptor mechanism or in the transmitting mechanism? One imagines that the only way of breaking out of the impasse is to invite a management consultancy firm to study our department, analyse what we are doing and, if possible, synthesise it into figures or simple words that even those who are reluctant to hear can understand. We seem to have tried all other measures and failed.

At last we have call-bells for each bed, at least in the main hospital. But has there been other upgrading of the wards with increased lavatory and washing amenity? In the exceptional summer of 1969 were many of the long-stay patients able to go into the grounds to enjoy the vitality-restoring sunshine? Unhappily the answers are negative to the last two questions. The kitty is bare and all these elemental top-priority things cannot be done. We have, however, literally some better beds, three of which are electrically operated.

There is a new millennium facing us—no longer this mirage, the Ten Year Plan. All the available monies of the region have poured into the building of a great new temple but four miles away from us. This is a joint venture, and the first of its kind, between the Medical Research Council and the Regional Hospital Board. Every plan or improvement has had to take its place in the queue and the reply to the starving asking for a dole of bread has not been the offer of cake, but 'wait for the opening of the new hospital'. All problems, the planners say publicly, will then be eased.

Privately they must have misgivings. Though even their private misgivings cannot equal a tenth of ours. We fear a regressive period. For years we have been the poor relation to the teaching hospitals in London—expected to provide a safety net for all who dropped out or off the teaching hospital conveyor belt system. That battle has been fought and the Regional Board has now won concession that each teaching hospital will undertake a territorial responsibility for the community round it. Miracle of miracles, some are even starting their own geriatric units. This can only augur well for the training of future generations of medical, nursing and ancillary staff.

No longer will happen what recently happened when we welcomed, for an afternoon visit, a group of final set nurses from a world-famous hospital. We started off by telling them of hopes for basic personal independence for each elderly patient. One of the lasses stopped us. Was she really comprehending aright? Did we really expect our patients to leave hospital? Yes. But they had understood from their tutor that they were spending the afternoon at a geriatric hospital? Nods of agreement came from the rest of the visiting party. "Yes," said the home team. Well surely patients never go out of geriatric hospitals except when dead?

The home team—forgetful that in this day and age such views could still exist—hastily shifted gear to direct the afternoon's discussion on different lines. It was a chastening experience. For here was a party of eager, intelligent, keen young women who, once they got on the same wavelength, were a joy and a stimulus to talk with. In such a small geographic area, how can such poor communication exist? One's thoughts revert to Chapter Eleven. "A rainbow and a cuckoo's song may never come together", but need this be so?

George Teeling-Smith,[1] Director of the Office of Health Economics, has reminded us that we cannot give the sort of help we ought to give to the elderly and the mentally handicapped and, at the same time, do all the kidney transplants. Although more money would help we will never solve the problem because we are going to find even more costly technical miracles to perform.

We are going to go on seeing a widening gap between technological and economic possibilities, the scope of medical support will extend in other ways also. Doctors are going to have to handle personal problems of families under their care.

We must, therefore, sit down sensibly and work out some system of priorities. The medical professions seem reluctant to do this and tend to work on a 'first come, first served basis', but there must be some sort of more rational process. This will only be brought about by expression of public concern and insistence, unless one is willing to wait for the time when the proportion of elderly in the population is as great and clamorous as the proportion of younger militants, and protesting mobs of the over-sixties sweep down Whitehall and sit-down in public buildings!

The Registrar-General predicts between 1971-1991 an overall increase in the total population of 16.8 per cent and in the age group 65-74 a rise of 6.8 per cent. The anticipated swell in the age group over 75 is predicted to be 35 per cent. This bulge is nearly upon us.

If this book ever goes into a third edition, the story may have taken a very different turn and mirror profound structural changes. Under the Green Paper plans, allied to the Redcliffe Maud report, our territorial area should be reduced to part of one Greater London Borough and a manageable total population. I would dare prophesy that the force of events will sweep ahead of the traditional, timorous piecemeal planning that seems to be the only emanation that reaches the ground-floor ear from the top floor. Community care will be a reality, there will be a revival of community initiative and sense of corporateness (the nearest an urban society can get to the old tribal interdependencies and modes of support); the so-called acute medicine and surgery will be carried out in small streamlined centres by highly technical professionals. We have already seen the astonishing decrease in need for obstetric beds by the use of hospital purely for the actual delivery and recovery and emergency period. This experience can be broadened to cover other areas.

We will probably find a need for more hostel or hotel-like accommodation to subserve the present hotel services that hospitals offer, but that should only be a temporary phase whilst housing development catches up and then perhaps surpasses the population needs. Grouped, warden-supported flatlets for the elderly and handicapped, adequate family accommodation and suitable provision for the lone single worker are not being planned or built in sufficient quantity. When there are enough, then the hotel function of hospitals will not be needed.

Given radical restructuring, perhaps we may yet have the opportunity to function as we wish and, as mentioned previously, in a new dimension helping to create new values, being a positive source of life norms and an active centre of humanism and giver of life as much as a possible saver. Or better still perhaps there will no longer be any need for such an anachronism as a Geriatric Department. Lines of demarcation will have faded and the rational process of being part of a community health team will at last come about.

> "Each individual carries in himself part of the
> social history of his time. He has been formed
> by his society and is helping to form it."
>
> *Enid Hutchinson*[2]

References

1. Teeling-Smith, George. *Hospital Times*. 26 July 1970.
2. Hutchinson, Enid. *Learning and Leisure in Middle and Later Life*. Pre-retirement Association. 1970.